# Essentials of Obstetrics and Gynaecology
# for
# Clinical Officers and Midwives

# Essentials of Obstetrics and Gynaecology
## for
# Clinical Officers and Midwives

## Vol. I: OBSTETRICS

## DR. JOHN N. K. MBILU

Writers Club Press

New York   Lincoln   Shanghai

Essentials of Obstetrics and Gynaecology
for Clinical Officers and Midwives
Vol. I: OBSTETRICS

Writers Club Press
an imprint of iUniverse, Inc.

For information address:
iUniverse
2021 Pine Lake Road, Suite 100
Lincoln, NE 68512
www.iuniverse.com

ISBN: 0-595-25646-5

Printed in the United States of America

This manual is dedicated to my parents, the late Mzee Naeman K. Mbilu and Otilie Mbilu.

"May God rest their Souls in Peace", Amen.

# CONTENTS

# FOREWORD

Dr. Mbilu must be congratulated on his sterling efforts in the production of such a book. This book describes the simple approach to the management of a woman during pregnancy, childbirth and postpartum period as well as her newborn infant.

The content contained in the chapters are what the author in his many years of obstetric practice, has found useful to be the guiding principles in the management of normal as well as "high risk" women during this critical period of their lives.

The basic elements in the book could be considered appropriate and useful in most situations in Guyana and many other developing countries when and if our available resources are effectively utilized. It is hoped that our Clinical Practitioners would make full use of this reference material when they seriously consider the welfare of our Maternal and Child Health (MCH) population, including the adolescents.

Dr. R. O. Cummings M.D; MPH
Chief Medical Officer.
Ministry of Health
Guyana.

# PREFACE

This book was written after many years of teaching Clinical Officers and Midwifery students Obstetrics and Gynaecology. The contents in this manual have helped many Clinical officers and Midwifery students in Tanzania and Guyana. This book has also helped Medical students of the University of Guyana as a revision book in preparation for their Qualifying final examinations. The students' constructive comments have been included in this book. It is my great hope that the book will be of use to Clinical Officers, Midwives and it will be a quick reference book for the medical personnel in the field. As it is difficult to include all the materials needed by students or field workers in one book, I make genuine request to other local Medical Workers to write more Health Learning Materials on this subject.

This Manual does not replace the classical renowned textbooks but it makes reading easier and quicker.

John N. K. Mbilu, MD; MMed

Consultant Obstetrician and Gynaecologist

Georgetown Guyana

# ACKNOWLEDGEMENTS

I would like to thank the staff of CEDHA Arusha, Tanzania, for helping to equip me with skills in book writing.

My thanks are also extended to Dr. W. K. Madundo, Dr. A. Janja, Dr. R. Kijangwa and Sr. Z. Nanyaro for having read the manual and given me constructive ideas. Many thanks go to the Clinical Officers and Midwifery students who encouraged me to prepare a manual for their use. I am indebted to Drs. M.Y. Bacchus, R. Luncheon, E. Hopkinson, R.O. Cummings, L. Lord, E. Sagala and C. Charles (Guyana) who contributed constructive comments after reviewing the manuscript, my thanks to them.

To Nurse-Midwives in Guyana, Ms. Joan Barry, Ms. Pauline Parris and Ms. Joyce Clarke, many thanks for being a part of the reviewing team. Also many special thanks to Ms. Byrnece Browne whose comments on reviewing the first draft enabled several adjustments to be made on this document.

Special thanks also go to Mr. Tyrone Doris, Ministry of Education (Guyana) who drew the illustrations.

I should also thank Dr. Sarah Gordon and Ms. Dawn Primo who supervised the word processing and printing of this book through the Health Learning Materials Unit, Ministry of Health (Annexe).

My acknowledgements would be incomplete without making mention of the Word Processing Clerks, Ms. Eraina Yaw, Ms. Omadel Charles

Ms. Marlyn Cozier and Ms. Carla James for their patience in typesetting this book.

My sincere thanks should also go to the publishers.

J.N.K.M

# CHAPTER 1

# ANATOMY OF THE FEMALE GENITAL TRACT

## INTRODUCTION

Knowledge of the anatomy of an organ or structure is the cornerstone of good medicine.

## OBJECTIVES

The student should be able to:
- Define genital tract.
- List the different organs of the female genital tract.
- Describe each of the genital organs in terms of appearance, blood supply, lymphatic drainage and functions.
- Draw and label the external genitalia of a female.
- Draw a sagittal section diagram of the uterus, cervix and vagina to show their relationship to the bladder, urethra and rectum.
- Describe the major uterine supports.

# DEFINITIONS

Genital organs are the organs of reproduction. In a female, there are external and internal genitalia.

# THE EXTERNAL FEMALE GENITALIA

## Vulva

The vulva is the female external genitalia, Fig.–11. The vulva is composed of:
- Mons pubis which is a cushion of fat lying over the pubic symphysis. The mons pubis is covered by skin and has hair in an adult woman.
- Labia major are two large folds of skin with fat. They are analogous to the male scrotum. The labia major are covered with hair in an adult woman. They contain apocrine, sebaceous and sweat glands.
- Labia minora are two thick skin folds that contain no fat or hair. The labia minor are homologous to the male penile urethra. The labia minor enclose the clitoris anteriorly. They also enclose the vagina and are fused posteriorly forming the fourchette.
- Vestibule is the space bounded by the labia minor. Within the vestibule are the external urethral meatus and the hymen.
- Clitoris is the structure which is homologous to the male penis. As the penis, the clitoris gets enlarged and stiffened during sexual excitement. The clitoris is about 2 cm long and is situated within the vestibule above the urethral meatus.
- Hymen is a thin and incomplete membrane covering the vaginal orifice in a virgin. The hymen has one or more openings. The hymeneal openings can be annular, crescent, septate or cribriform.

The hymeneal openings allow menstrual blood to escape during menstruation. The hymen is torn during intercourse and/or child-birth. The tags of a torn hymen are known as "carunculae myrti-formes." A woman with an intact hymen is said to be virgin.

- Bartholin's glands lie beneath the labia major and open on the inner side of labia minor. They lubricate the vagina. The Bartholin's ducts are homologous to the male Cowper's ducts.

## Vulval blood supply

The vulva is highly vascularised. It gets its blood supply from:
- Vaginal artery which is a branch of the internal iliac artery.
- Superficial pudendal artery which is a branch of the femoral artery.

## Vulval lymphatic drainage, see Fig.–2

The main drainage site of the vulva is the superficial inguinal lymph nodes. The lymphatic drainage extends to the deep inguinal lymph nodes then to the external iliac lymph nodes and the common iliac lymph nodes. There is a contra-lateral lymphatic drainage of the labia.

# THE INTERNAL FEMALE GENITALIA

## Vagina

The vagina is a tube-like passage connecting the vulva and the uterus. The vaginal wall is lined with rugae, which allow it to expand during sexual intercourse and childbirth. The vagina is always moist, the fluid being derived from cervical secretions and Bartholin's glands. This fluid has an acidic reaction making it capable of resisting infection. The vagina is divided into four areas in relation to the cervix. The four vaginal areas are called fornices.

- Anterior fornix is the shallowest of the fornices; measuring about 9 cm in an adult female.
- Posterior fornix is the deepest of all fornices; measuring about 11 cm in an adult female.
- Two lateral fornices.

The relationship of the vagina to the surrounding organs is as shown in Fig.–3.

> Anteriorly there is the urethra and urinary bladder.
> Posteriorly there is the perineal body, rectum and the peritoneum of the Pouch of Douglas.
> Laterally there are the sphincter vaginae, levator ani muscles, lateral fornices and Bartholin's glands.
> Superiorly is the cervix.

## Vaginal blood supply

The vagina gets its blood supply from the vaginal artery, branches of the pudendal artery and twigs from the middle and inferior rectal arteries.

## Vaginal lymphatic drainage

The lower one third of the vagina has the same lymphatic drainage as that of the vulva while the upper two thirds has the same lymphatic drainage as that of the cervix.

# THE UTERUS

The uterus is a hollow pear-shaped thick-walled muscular organ. In an adult female it measures about 9 cm long, 3 cm, thick and 6 cm broad at its widest part. The cavity of the uterus is lined by a columnar epithelium called endometrium. The uterus is divided into three (3) main parts, Fig.–4.

- The fundus is the part above the insertion of the fallopian tubes.
- The body is the middle portion of the uterus.
- The cervix (Fig.–5) is the lowest portion of the uterus, which projects into the vagina. It is divided into two parts; the supra-vaginal and infra-vaginal (portio-vaginalis) portions. The cervix has a canal, which opens into the uterine cavity at the internal os and into the vagina at the external os. The external os of a nulli-parous cervix is circular while that of a multiparous is a transverse slit. The cervix is made up of more connective tissue (80%) than muscle while the body has more muscle (80%) than connective tissue.

The normal anatomical position of the uterus is anteflexion and anteversion. The peritoneum is reflected from the bladder over the front of the uterus where it becomes adherent to the uterus. Posterior to the uterus, the peritoneum forms the Pouch of Douglas and anteriorly the utero-vesical pouch.

The relationship of the uterus to its surrounding organs is as shown in Fig.–3.

- ➤ Anteriorly there is the utero-vesical peritoneum and the urinary bladder.
- ➤ Posteriorly there is the Pouch of Douglas and coils of intestines.
- ➤ Superiorly there are coils of the intestines and omentum.
- ➤ Inferiorly is the hymen.
- ➤ Laterally is the parametrium.

# Blood supply of the uterus

The uterus gets its main blood supply from the uterine artery, which is a branch of the internal iliac artery. The ovarian artery, which is a branch of the abdominal aorta, also nourishes the uterus. The two arteries anastomose along the fallopian tube.

## Uterine supports

The uterine supports, which prevent the uterus from prolapsing, are in pairs, Fig.–6.

- The cardinal ligaments, also known as the transverse cervical or Mackenrod's ligaments. These are the strongest of all the uterine supports.
- Utero-sacral ligaments.
- Pubo-cervical ligaments are the weakest.

Apart from the above listed ligaments there are other ligaments, the round ligaments (prevent the uterus from axial rotation and maintain its ante-flexion state) and the broad ligaments through which the blood vessels nourishing the uterus and fallopian tubes pass. The levator ani muscles, which act as pelvic floor support and prevent the uterus from prolapsing.

## Fallopian tubes

There are two fallopian tubes, each of which measures about 10–20 cm long. Each fallopian tube is divided into three major parts, Fig.–7.

- Interstitial portion is the part of fallopian tube which is within the uterine muscle. This interstitial portion opens into the uterine cavity. It is the narrowest part of the fallopian tube.
- The isthmus is the middle part of the tube.
- The ampulla is the widest trumpet-like part of the fallopian tube. The end of the ampulla has finger-like projections known as fimbriae.

Blood supply of the fallopian tube is like that of the uterus.

## OVARIES

There are two ovaries, one on each side of the uterus, Fig.–7. The ovaries are oval shaped and attached to the uterus by the ovarian ligament. The ovarian artery supplies each ovary. They produce ova and steroid hormones (progesterone and oestrogen).

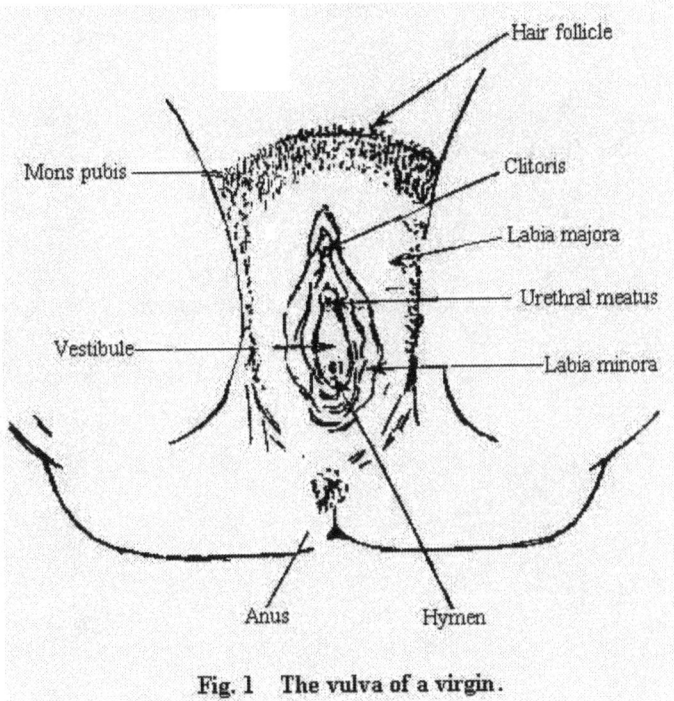

Fig. 1   **The vulva of a virgin.**

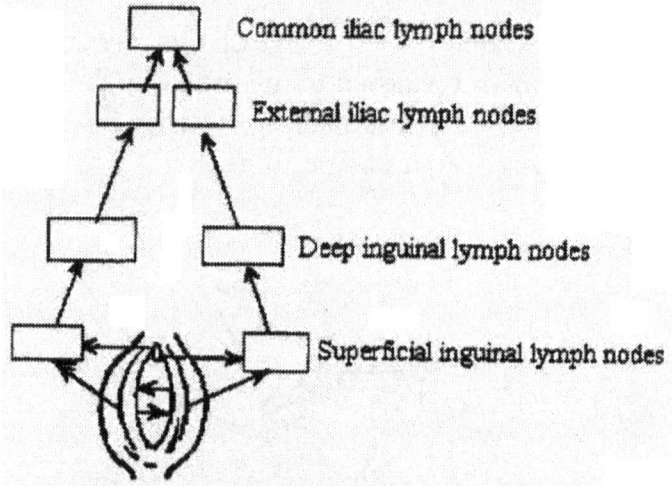

Fig. 2   Lymphatic drainage of the vulva.

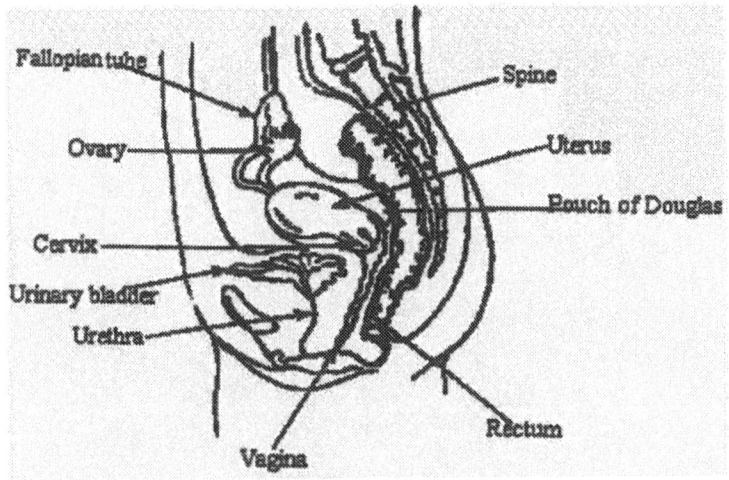

**Fig. 3 Sagittal view of female reproductive tract.**

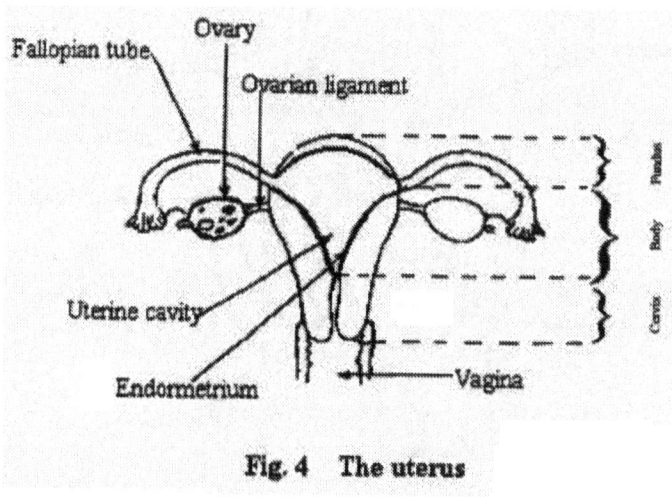

**Fig. 4    The uterus**

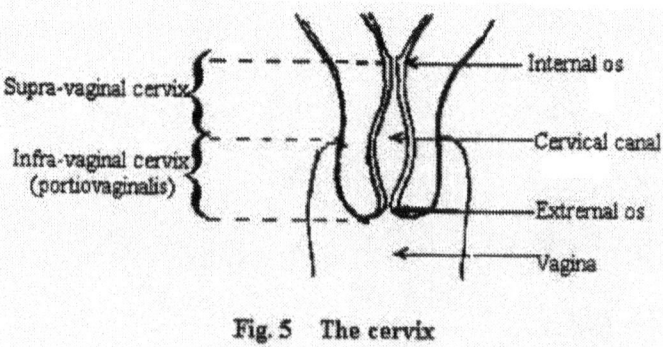

**Fig. 5    The cervix**

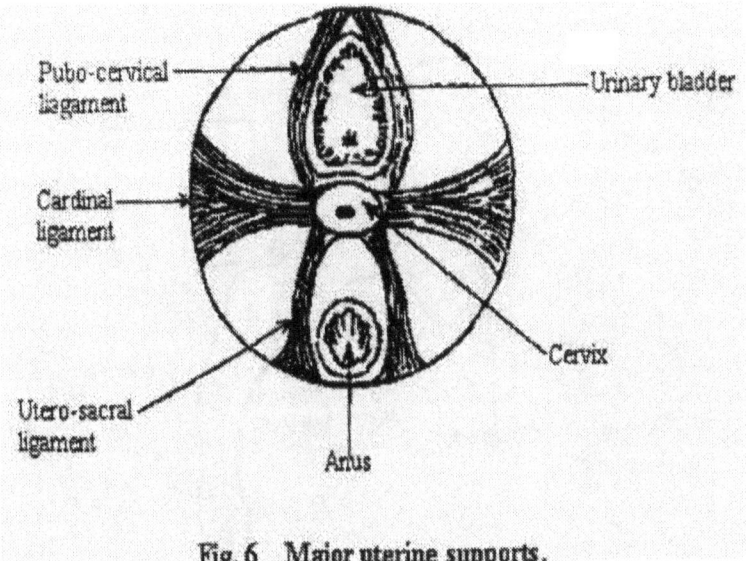

**Fig. 6   Major uterine supports.**

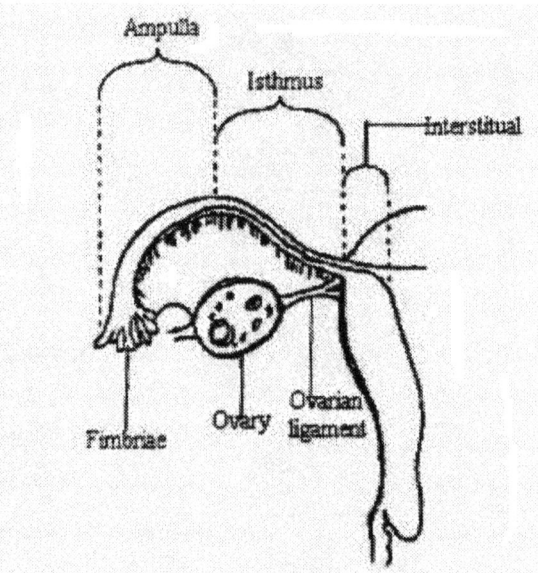

**Fig. 7   The fallopian tube (left side not shown).**

# CHAPTER 2

# OBSTETRIC ANATOMY

## INTRODUCTION

So as to predict the outcome of labour, knowledge of the anatomy of the pelvis, foetal skull and the uterus is paramount.

## OBJECTIVES

The student should be able to:
- Draw and label the female pelvic bones.
- Identify on a bone or diagram the main landmarks of the pelvis.
- Name the diameters of the pelvis.
- Perform pelvic assessment in a pregnant woman.
- Identify a normal pelvis.
- Draw and label a foetal skull.

## THE FEMALE PELVIS

### Anatomy of the female pelvis

The female pelvis is made up of four bones joined at three points, Fig.–1.

- The innominate bones are two bones formed by three bones (ilium, pubis and ischium) which join completely at puberty. The innominate bones are on the antero-lateral aspect of the pelvis.
- Sacrum is wedge-shaped and made up of five fused sacral vertebrae. The upper part of the first sacral vertebra and lower part of the fifth lumbar vertebra form the sacral promontory of the sacrum. The sacrum forms the posterior aspect of the pelvis. The sacrum is slightly curved to allow and to accommodate the foetus during its passage.
- The coccyx forms the tail end of the spine. It has 4–5 fine fused bones.

The bony pelvis is divided into false pelvis, formed by the flaring ilia, (this has less obstetrical significance) and the true pelvis.

## Parts of the true pelvis

The true pelvis has:
- Pelvic inlet which is the plane of the pelvic brim. The inlet is bounded by the pubis interiorly, the alae and sacral promontory posteriorly and the ileo-pectineal line laterally. The antero-posterior diameter of the inlet is about 11.0 cm and the transverse diameter is about 13.0 cm.
- The mid cavity is bounded by the pelvic brim above, the plane of the outlet below, the sacrum posteriorly, laterally by the ligaments sacrotuberous and ischial bones, anteriorly by the obturator foramen, ascending rami of ischia and the pubis, Fig.–9. The diameter is about 12 cm all round.
- The outlet of the pelvis, roughly triangular in shape, is bounded anteriorly by the pubic arch, posteriorly by the tip of coccyx and laterally by the sacrotuberous ligaments and ischial tuberosities.

The transverse diameter of the outlet is about 11 cm and the antero-posterior diameter is about 13 cm.

## Assessment of the pelvis

Clinically the pelvis is assessed during pregnancy at 37–38 weeks of gestation and during labour so as to predict the possibility of vaginal delivery of the foetus. Pelvic assessment should be done aseptically.

The patient is placed in a dorsal position with her legs fully flexed and abducted. The patient should be reassured that the procedure is painless. The examiner wears a sterile glove in his/her right hand and cleans the perineum with antiseptic. The index and middle fingers of the gloved hand are lubricated with cream. The two fingers are introduced into the vagina towards the sacro-promontory. The examining hand is then rotate so as to palpate the ischial spines. Then the hand is rotated back to its first position and starting from the sacro-promontory the fingers are swept over the sacral curve. After reaching the end of the coccyx the examining hand is rotated anteriorly and the examining fingers are pushed into the pubic angle. Then the examining hand is withdrawn from the vagina and clenched. The knuckles of the clenched fist are pushed between the ischial tuberosities.

## Characteristics of an ideal obstetric pelvis

An ideal obstetric pelvis should have the following dimensions:
- The sacral-promontory should not be reached. Clinically this measures the diagonal diameter, the lower border of the symphysis pubis to the sacral promontory, which is approximately 11.5 cm.
- The ischial spines should not be prominent.
- The pubic angle should admit two fingers (approximately 85–90°).

- The intertuberous diameter should admit four knuckles (approximately 10.0 cm).

# THE FOETAL SKULL

The foetal skull has five important bones on its vault, Fig.–10. From front to back are two frontal bones, two parietal bones and one occipital bone. The foetal skull bones are separated by sutures as shown in Fig.–10. The sutures meet at the fontanelles.

- The anterior fontanelle is rhomboid in shape and joins four sutures, two coronary, one sagittal and one frontal suture.
- The posterior fontanelle is triangular in shape and joins three sutures, two lambdoid and one sagittal suture.

The foetal skull is divided into four regions which aid the description of the presenting part of the foetus as palpated per vaginum during labour.

- ➢ The occiput is the area lying behind the posterior fontanelle.
- ➢ The bregma is the area of the anterior fontanelle.
- ➢ The vertex is the area lying between the two parietal eminences, the anterior and posterior fontanelle.
- ➢ The sinciput is the area in front of the anterior fontanelle. The sinciput is further divided into the brow (the area between the anterior fontanelle and the root of the nose) and the face, (the area below the root of the nose; and the tip of the chin).

## Foetal skull diameters Figure–11

The diameters shown are for the possible presentation of the foetal skull.

- Sub-occipito-bregmatic is from the nape of the neck to the centre of the bregma. This diameter is about 9.5 cm long. It is the diameter of vertex presentation.
- Mento-vertical is from tip of the chin to above the posterior fontanelle. This diameter is about 14.0 cm and is the diameter for brow presentation.
- Sub-mento-bregmatic is from centre of bregma to below the chin. It is about 9.5 cm. It is the diameter for face presentation when the chin is pointing upwards, that is mento-anterior. In mento-posterior the diameter is sterno-bregmatic that is from the bregma to the upper border of the sternum. Sterno-bregmatic diameter is about 18.0 cm long.
- Occipito-frontal is from the root of the nose to the occiput. It is about 11.0 cm. It is the diameter of the vertex in occiput-posterior position.

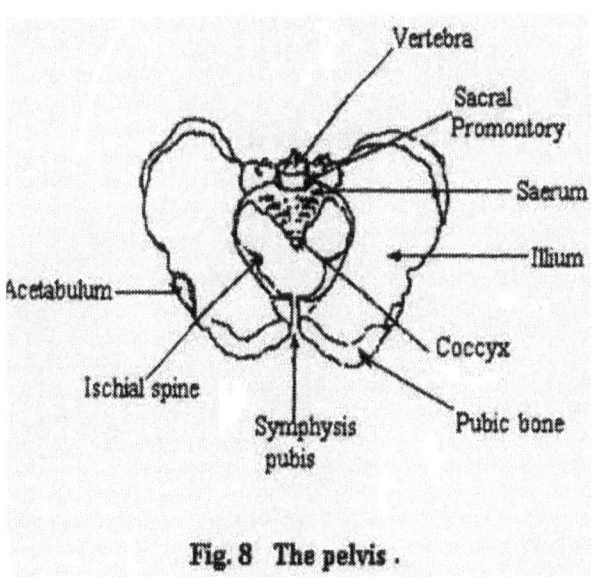

**Fig. 8 The pelvis .**

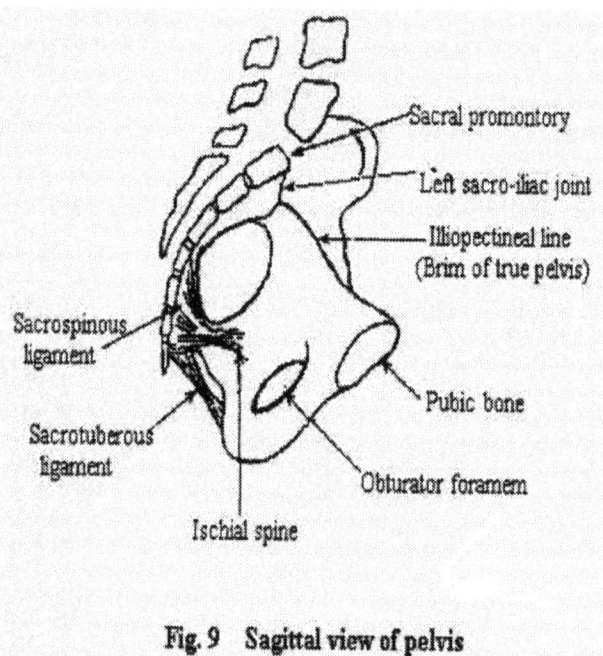

**Fig. 9   Sagittal view of pelvis**

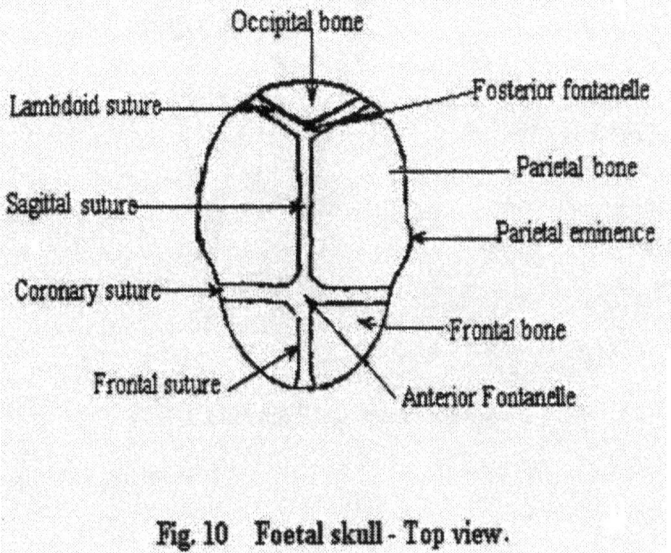

Fig. 10    Foetal skull - Top view.

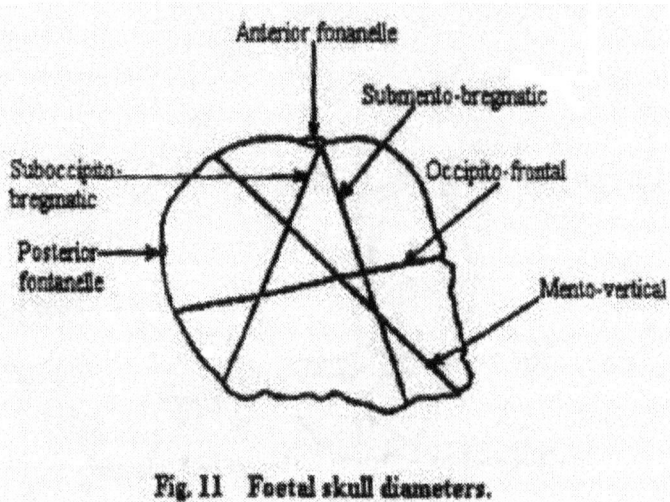

**Fig. 11    Foetal skull diameters.**

# CHAPTER 3

# FERTILIZATION AND PLACENTATION

## INTRODUCTION

Embryology is too vast a subject to be dealt fully in such a small book.

## OBJECTIVES

The student is expected to be able to:
- Define fertilization.
- Describe briefly the process of fertilization, embryo formation and placentation.
- Describe the anatomy of the placenta.
- List at least four types of placental malformation.
- List the functions of the placenta.

## FERTILIZATION

### Definition

Fertilization (conception) means the union of a sperm and an ovum.

# The process of fertilization

The sperms can only pass through the cervical canal and get into the uterine cavity and through the fallopian tubes during ovulation time. During ovulation period there is a change in the cervical mucus which allows the sperms to penetrate through the cervical canal. The ovum extruded from the ovary at the time of ovulation is picked up by the fimbriae of the fallopian tube. The ovum is propelled through the tube into the uterine cavity by the help of hair processes of the tube combined with its peristalsis. Normally the union of the ovum and sperm takes place in the ampulla portion of the tube. Usually only one sperm is necessary for fertilizing one ovum. For fertilization to take place the man concerned has to have a normal spermatogram characterized by:

- Amount of ejaculum should be 2–5 mls.
- Sperm count range should be 20–60 million per ml (a few fertile men have smaller counts but should not be less than 10 million per ml).
- Morphology. About 80% of the sperms should be normal.
- Viscosity of the ejaculum should be normal.
- Motility. About 60% of the sperms should have forward movement.

After ejaculation all sperms that remain in the vagina for more than two hours are killed as the vaginal environment is acidic. The sperms which enter the cervical canal, within a few minutes after ejaculation, retain their fertility as the cervical environment is alkaline.

After 48 hours sperms lose their fertility while for ovum it takes 24 hours. Fertilization is therefore possible if coitus takes place within 48 hours before ovulation or within 24 hours after ovulation. This means if ovulation occurs on the 14th day of a menstrual cycle, fertilization can take place after sexual intercourse on the 12th, 13th, 14th and 15th day.

# ZYGOTE IMPLANTATION AND EMBRYO FORMATION

The fertilized ovum (zygote) takes 3–4 days to travel through the fallopian tube and reaches the uterine cavity by the 7$^{th}$ day from ovulation. It is fully embedded (implanted) into the endometrium by the 14$^{th}$ day (just at the time when the next menstrual cycle is expected).

While the zygote is in the fallopian tube it divides repeatedly to form a round mass of cells called morula. The morula develops into a blastocyst with an outer cell layer called the trophoblast. It starts to embed into the endometrium on the 7$^{th}$ day from ovulation. The trophoblast produces hormones similar to lutinizing hormone (L.H.) which directs the corpus luteum to persist until 12 weeks of gestation when the placenta is matured enough to take over all the hormonal production necessary to maintain the pregnancy. The trophoblast also produces HCG (Human Chorionic Gonadotrophin). The blastocyst has an inner cell mass which differentiates into two distinct masses: an outer or ectodermal layer and an inner or endodermal layer. Further differentiation produces a third layer between the endoderm and the ectoderm called mesoderm. The combination of trophoblast and mesoderm forms a chorion. The mesoderm, ectoderm and endoderm are the primitive cells from which embryogenesis takes place. The ectoderm later gives rise to formation of the nervous system, the medulla of adrenal gland, skin and its appendages, and other glands like the pituitary and salivary glands. The endoderm forms the gastro-intestinal tract, liver, gall-bladder, biliary tract, pancreas, respiratory system and germ cells of gonads. The mesoderm forms the bones, muscles, cartilage, connective tissues, serous lining, cardio-vascular system and most of the genital tract.

The embryonic stage is completed by the end of the 8th week of gestation and thereafter it is called a foetus.

# THE PLACENTA

## Placentation

At first chorionic villi are present all around the blastocyst, but later they atrophy on the side adjacent to the uterine cavity and persist on the side adjacent to the uterine wall. The side of the blastocyst without chorionic villi forms the chorionic laeve while the part with the villi is the chorionic frondosum. The chorionic frondosum further develops to form the placenta, which is connected to the foetus by the umbilical cord. By the 12th week of gestation the placenta is fully formed and takes over the functions of the corpus luteum.

## Anatomy of the placenta

A fully formed placenta is disc-like and weighs about 500 gms. The maternal side of the placenta is dark-red and divided into 15–20 segments called cotyledons. The foetal side of the placenta is covered by amnionic and chorionic membranes.

The umbilical cord has two arteries and one vein embedded in Wharton's jelly. The Wharton's jelly is a loose myxomatous tissue of mesodermal origin. The jelly acts as a physical buffer and prevents kinking of the cord and interference of blood circulation.

## Functions of the placenta

The placenta is an important organ for the life of the foetus. The placenta has many functions:

- The placenta is an organ of respiration for the foetus. Oxygen from the mother diffuses into the foetus through the placenta and carbon dioxide from the foetus diffuses through the placenta into the maternal blood circulation.
- The placenta forms a barrier between the foetus and the mother.
- The placenta is an organ of excretion for the foetus.
- Nutrients like glucose and amino acids are transferred from the mother to the foetus through the placenta.
- The placenta produces hormones like oestrogen, progesterone, human chorionic gonadotrophin and human placental lactogen which maintain the pregnancy.

The placenta thus maintains and nourishes the growing foetus.

## Abnormalities of the placenta

A variety of abnormalities of the placenta can occur, such as:
- Abnormalities of implantation. Normally the placenta is situated in the upper segment of the body and more commonly at the fundus. If the placenta touches or is implanted in the lower segment this is abnormal (see chapter on A.P.H.).
- Abnormal insertion of the umbilical cord. Usually the umbilical cord enters the placenta at its midpoint. Marginal insertion of the cord (battledore placenta) is a rare variation. The umbilical vessels may run for some distance through the membranes before entering the placenta called velamentous insertion.
- Extra placenta. There could be an extra placental lobe called succenturiate lobe or the placenta may be divided into two separate lobes but united by primary vessels and membranes called bipartite placenta.
- Adherent placenta. Placenta accreta (the chorionic villi attached onto the myometrial cells), placenta increta (the chorionic villi

penetrate the myometrium to some degree) and placenta percreta (the chorionic villi penetrate the serosal surface of the uterus).

- Placenta membranacea. Here the chorion laeve has not atrophied thus the villi are maintained. This happens when the decidua capsularis is so well vascularised.

# CHAPTER 4

# NORMAL PREGNANCY

## INTRODUCTION

In an ordinary antenatal clinic, about 90% of the clients have normal pregnancies. The midwife in the antenatal clinic should make sure that her client carries a normal pregnancy to delivery.

## OBJECTIVES

The student should be able to:
- Define a normal pregnancy.
- Define some of the commonly used terms for a pregnant woman.
- Calculate the gestation period by dates and expected date of delivery.
- Determine the age of the pregnancy by fundal palpation.
- Diagnose pregnancy.
- Discuss the normal physiological changes in a pregnant woman.

# DEFINITION OF NORMAL PREGNANCY

A pregnancy is said to be normal if it grows as expected, the foetus is lying longitudinally with vertex presentation and the woman is well physically and mentally.

# DEFINITION OF COMMON TERMS

In order for the student to be able to communicate with other staff in the antenatal clinic or labour ward he/she should know some of the commonly used terms:

- Gravida refers to a uterus with pregnancy. The gravidity does not matter whether the pregnancy ended in an abortion, ectopic, stillbirth or live birth. For example a woman is pregnant and this pregnancy is her fourth thus she the woman is not pregnant at the time of seeing her, she is Gravida 0 even if she had previous pregnancies.
- Parity means that there has occurred a delivery of a baby from the gestation parity. If the woman had a multiple pregnancy and delivers the babies then each baby carries its own parity. If the woman had either an abortion or ectopic pregnancy then the number of such pregnancies is added to the parity as illustrated in the following examples:
  - ➤ A woman is pregnant for the fourth time and she delivered three times. In the first pregnancy the baby died one month after delivery ; the second pregnancy she had a stillbirth and the third delivery was a normal and healthy baby, this woman is said to be Gravida 4 Para 3. If the same woman had twins in a previous pregnancy then she is said to be Gravida 4 Para 4.
  - ➤ If the same woman had an abortion (or ectopic) in her first pregnancy, a live baby in her second pregnancy and in her

third pregnancy she had another live baby she is said to be Gravida 4 Para 2+1; the +1 number refers to the abortion (or ectopic).
- Primigravida refers to a woman who is pregnant for the first time.
- Primipara refers to a woman who had one delivery only.
- Multigravida refers to a woman carrying the second or more pregnancy. This is true whether the previous pregnancies ended with an abortion, ectopic, stillbirth or live child.
- Multipara refers to a woman who had two or more viable deliveries that is a pregnancy carried to at least 24 weeks.

# DETERMINING THE GESTATION PERIOD

The duration of a normal pregnancy is 280 days (40 weeks or 10 lunar months or 9 calendar months), counting from the first day of the last normal menstrual period (LMP). If counting starts from the time of ovulation, the duration of pregnancy is 266 days.

The Expected Date of Delivery (EDD) is commonly counted from the LMP using either of the following formulae:
- Add 7 days to the date, subtract 3 months from the month and add one to the year of the LMP.
  For Example: LMP = 04/ 05/2000
  $$EDD = 04(+7)/05(-3)/2000(+1)$$
  $$= 11/02/2001$$
- Add 7 to the date add 9 to the month and add 0 to the year of the LMP.
  For example: LMP = 04/09/2000
  $$EDD = 04(+7)/05(+9)/2000(+0)$$
  $$= 11/14/2000$$
  $$= 1102/2001$$

If the patient does not remember the exact date when she had her LMP then she should be asked if she had it during the early, mid or late part of the month and then the EDD is calculated from the estimates.

> THE LMP OF A PREGNANT WOMAN SHOULD ALWAYS BE ESTABLISHED.

# DIAGNOSIS OF PREGNANCY

## Symptoms of pregnancy

- Amenorrhoea means the absence of menstruation. Amenorrhoea is the first and commonest symptom of pregnancy.

> AN AMENORRHOEIC WOMAN DURING HER REPRODUCTIVE AGE IS PREGNANT UNLESS PROVED OTHERWISE.

Sometimes a woman might notice spotting or scanty vaginal bleeding during embryo implantation (implantation haemorrhage) or get reduced vaginal bleeding in the first three months of pregnancy. This bleeding might make the patient and the midwife think that there is no amenorrhoea thus the last normal period, should be the only one considered

> A DETAILED MENSTRUAL HISTORY IS IMPORTANT.

- Morning sickness is characterized by nausea and/or vomiting and salivation. The vomiting is usually in the morning but it can happen during other times of the day.
- Breasts become heavy and painful due to engorgement.

- Loss of appetite and dislike of certain foods. Extraordinary taste for odd things like sand and charcoal.
- Constitutional symptoms include depressive states, fatigue and feeling of heaviness.
- Frequency of micturation due to compression of the bladder by the uterus.
- Quickening is the feeling of foetal movements by the mother. Quickening begins at 18–20 weeks of gestation in primigravidae while it is earlier (16–18 weeks) in multigravidae.

## Signs of pregnancy

- Breast changes. The breasts are engorged, tender and secrete clear fluid. The areola is blackened and has Montgomeroy's tubercles.
- Colour change. The woman might develop black patches (chloasma) and linea nigra (a black line extending from the pubic symphysis to the xiphoid process). This blackening colour change on the skin is due to an excessive deposit of melanin.
- Striae gravidarum. Irregular, linear, pink to purple, slightly depressed, finely wrinkled stripes in the skin of the abdomen, buttocks, breasts and thighs. Striae gravidarum are due to weakening of the collagenous or elastic fibres and loss of the ground substance in the subdermal tissues. Striae can also occur in cases of obesity, Cushing's syndrome and Addison's disease.
- Bluish vaginal wall (Jacquemeir's sign). There is also increased pulsation in the lateral fornices (Osiander's sign).
- Growing of the uterine fundus:
  - ➤ 12 weeks, the fundus is just palpable at the upper border of the pubic symphysis.
  - ➤ 14 weeks, the fundus is between the 16 week's level and the pubic symphysis.

- ➤ 16 weeks, the fundus is midway between the pubic symphysis and the umbilicus.
- ➤ 18 week, the fundus is two fingers below the umbilicus.
- ➤ 20 weeks, the fundus is at the level of the umbilicus.
- ➤ 24 weeks the fundus is between the 28 week's level and the umbilicus.
- ➤ 28 weeks, the fundus is between the xiphoid process and the umbilicus.
- ➤ 34 week, the fundus is between the tip of the xiphoid process and the 28 week's level.
- ➤ 36 weeks, the fundus is at the tip of the xiphoid process.
- ➤ 38 and 40 weeks, the fundus is two fingers below the xiphoid process. The reduction in fundal height between 38–40 weeks is as a result of "lightening". Lightening is due to the decrease of amniotic fluid. Also descent of the presenting part of the foetus causes decrease in fundal height.

The estimation of the duration of pregnancy by using the first mentioned body landmarks is more exact up to 20 weeks gestation, thereafter the estimates are not very reliable.

The duration of pregnancy can also be estimated by using finger-breadths (the middle three fingers only). Above the umbilicus a finger's breath is equal to two weeks, while below the umbilicus it is equal to one week.

The fundal height can also be measured by a tape measure. The tape measurement is better than the other methods, mentioned above, as it is reproducible and has fewer observer errors. The height in centimetres is equivalent to the gestation period in the first 20 weeks there after a conversion factor or a percentile graph (as shown below) should be used.

# Uterine height graph

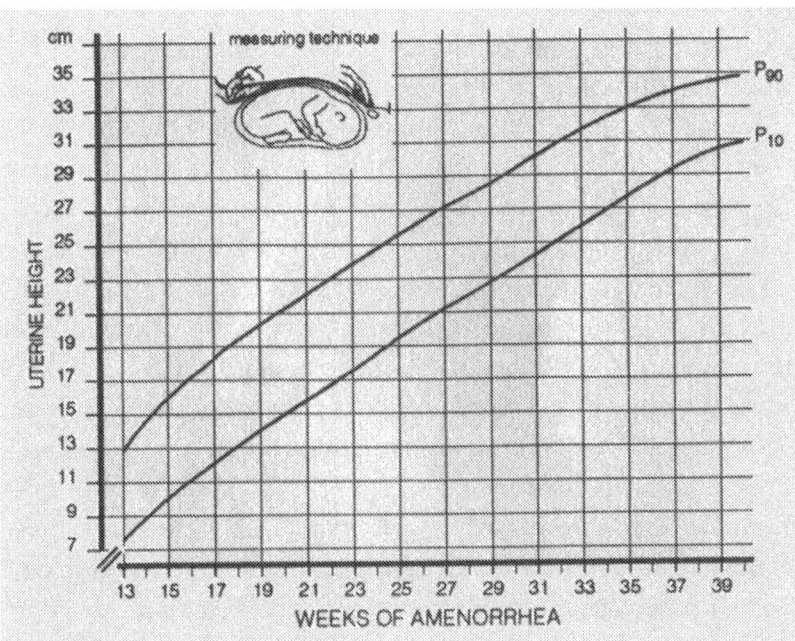

- Foetal heart sounds start to be audible by using a mono-aural foetal stethoscope (Pinard type) from 24 weeks. The foetal heart sound rate is between 120–160/min. The foetal heart should be distinguished from the maternal pulse transmitted by the aorta or the uterine artery (uterine soufflé). The foetal heart is faster and asynchronous to the maternal pulse. The foetal heart can be heard earlier with more sensitive equipments like daptone (12 weeks) and ultrasound (7 weeks).

## Investigations

Investigations that can be done at a Health centre to prove the presence of pregnancy include

- Pregnancy tests. The test available in health centre uses the agglutination-inhibition principle. The reagent used is plumose. Principally the test detects the presence of Human Chorionic Gondotrophin (HCG) produced by the placenta and excreted in the urine. The planosec contains two plates, one of which contains latex coated with human HCG and the other contains anti-HCG serum. If urine of a non-pregnant woman is mixed with antisera and then mixed with the latex there will be agglutination; this is a NEGATIVE test. If the urine contains HCG and is treated in the same way then there will not be agglutination; this is a POSITIVE test. The planosec will only be positive six weeks from the LMP and not earlier.
- Enzyme linked immunosorbant assay (ELISA) are now commercially available. The essay depends on the double reaction of standard phase antibody with enzyme labelled antibody which is sensitive and so able to detect very low HCG. The positive results can be detected as early as 10 days after fertilisation that is about four days before the first menstrual period.
- Abdominal X-ray taken after 16 weeks of pregnancy will show foetal skeleton. X-raying a pregnant woman is not advisable, for the X-rays might damage the gonads of both the mother and the foetus. Also leukaemia is more common in children who had been X-rayed in-utero. This investigation is not recommended due to the listed complications.
- Other tests like ultrasonography and blood immunoassays.

# NORMAL PHYSIOLOGICAL CHANGES IN A PREGNANT WOMAN

Though pregnancy is not a disease, a pregnant woman has some physiological changes that are due to her pregnancy state and are normal.

## Body weight

During pregnancy the woman's body weight increases by 25% of her non-pregnant state. The body weight increases at the average of 0.5 kg per week (ranging from 0.2 0.9 kg per week), thus she will increase a total of about 12.5 kg by the time she delivers. The increase in weight is due to:

- The growing foetus. The average weight of a newborn baby is 3.4 kg.
- Enlargement of maternal organs like the uterus and breasts.
- The maternal deposition of adipose tissues.
- The increase in maternal blood volume and total body fluid.

## Metabolism in pregnancy

Pregnancy is a catabolic condition. The metabolism increases in pregnancy largely due to the foetus. In advanced pregnancy, energy requirement is approximately 2,500 cal per day (in non-pregnant 2,100 cal per day). During lactation there is further energy increase to 3,000 cal per day due to milk production. There is thus a rise in basal metabolic rate due to increased oxygen consumption. To maintain the increased total metabolism there is an increased activity in control mechanisms:

- The anterior pituitary secretes more thyroid stimulating hormone (TSH).
- The thyroid gland hypertrophies and is enlarged in about 70% of the women. The enlarged thyroid extracts iodine from the blood more effectively and the serum content is reduced. The protein

bound iodine (PBI) is increased to 8–10mg/dl (non-pregnant level is 5–6 mg/dl).

- Carbohydrate metabolism is increased. During pregnancy there are increased insulin antagonists (oestrogen, progesterone, corticosteroid and human placental lactogen). Insulinase produced by the placenta destroys insulin. As the insulin is the main hormone regulating glucose metabolism, blood sugar circulates for a longer time in the maternal blood. The circulation of sugar in the maternal blood stream is advantageous to the foetus, which depends on the maternal glucose. Pregnancy is thus a diabetogenic state. Diabetes mellitus can thus appear or be worsened during pregnancy. Due to the increase in blood sugar, glycosuria is common during pregnancy.
- Protein intake and absorption is increased during pregnancy. There is reduced amino acid metabolism. The blood urea in a pregnant woman is 10–15 mg/dl (non-pregnant level is 20–40 mg/dl).
- Fat is stored as fatty tissue.

## Respiratory changes during pregnancy

During pregnancy there is hyperventilation. The hyperventilation causes increase in oxygen intake and carbon dioxide output. The maternal blood has thus high oxygen concentration and low carbon dioxide concentration. This difference in gas concentration in the maternal blood makes oxygen supply to the foetus from the mother possible and the transfer of carbon dioxide from the foetus to the maternal blood easy.

## Cardiovascular changes during pregnancy

Pregnancy causes a physiological burden to the heart due to:
- Increased oxygen demand:

- ➤ The foetus consumes more oxygen per unit volume then the mother.
- ➤ Most of the maternal tissues are hypertrophied and their oxygen demand is thus increased.
- ➤ Increased muscular work of moving her increased size and that of the foetus.
- Increased blood volume. During pregnancy the total blood volume increases by about 40–50%.
- Increased mechanical disadvantage due to the enlarged maternal uterus.
  - ➤ The heart is displaced upwards and rotated to the right.
  - ➤ The heart is splinted to the diaphragm.
- Increased cardiac output by about 30%. It reaches maximum between 24–32 weeks of pregnancy. Cardiac output also increases by 30% at the height of the mother's bearing down efforts during labour. The pulse rate also increases.

## Urinary system changes during pregnancy

The renal blood flow is increased by about 40%. The glomerular filtration rate is also increased by 40%. Due to increased oestrogen concentrations the muscles of the bladder and ureters are relaxed.

- Increased frequency of micturation due to:
  - ➤ Increased urine production.
  - ➤ Maternal compression of the uterus by the uterus;
    - ✓ Early in pregnancy as the uterus comes out of the pelvis.
    - ✓ Later in pregnancy as the foetal head descends into the pelvis.
    - ✓ During micturation especially when the woman assumes the squatting position.
- Hydro-ureters. This is due to:

> ➤ Oestrogen causing relaxation of the ureters and decreased peristalsis.
> ➤ Compression of the ureters by the enlarged uterus.

The above can cause stasis of urine and thus bacterial proliferation and development of urinary tract infection is more likely to occur during pregnancy.

• Reduced renal threshold particularly to glucose. This can lead to glycosuria.

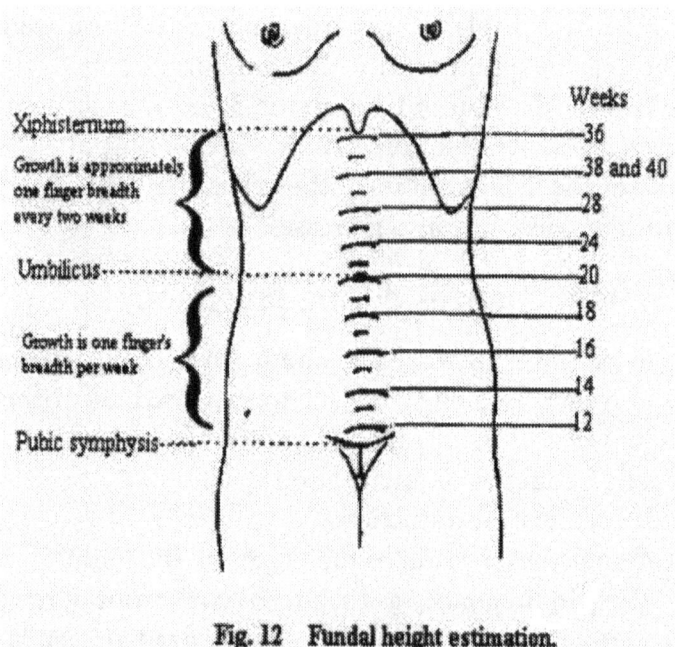

**Fig. 12  Fundal height estimation.**

# CHAPTER 5

# MINOR AILMENTS OF PREGNANCY

## INTRODUCTION

Pregnancy is not a disease, but it is true to say that a pregnant woman does not feel as normal as when not pregnant! There are some pregnancy related complaints which, when excessive, need to be treated. Most of the common minor ailments can be treated at a health centre.

## OBJECTIVES

The student is expected to be able to:
- List the common minor ailments of pregnancy.
- Diagnose and treat minor ailments of pregnancy.
- Diagnose and manage Hyperemesis gravidarum.

## MORNING SICKNESS

About 50% of women experience nausea and or vomiting of minor degree in early pregnancy up to the fourteenth week of pregnancy. The woman can vomit early in the morning or any other time. Some women experience excessive salivation. The cause of this condition is not known but it could be due to high levels of human chorionic gonadotrophins. In some women morning sickness is made worse by certain odours of foods like fatty foods.

Morning sickness can interfere with the patient's nutrition. The patient should be advised to take small amounts of food, frequently. She should avoid heavy meals or staying for a long time hungry or eating fatty food as all these can increase nausea. The patient should also be advised to drink a lot of fluids. If the condition is very disturbing anti-emetic like promethazine (25 mg six hourly), dimenhydrinate (gravol 50mg six hourly) and chlorpheniramine (4 mg six hourly) can be given by injection or orally.

Morning sickness improves spontaneously by the 14$^{th}$ or 16$^{th}$ week of pregnancy.

# HYPEREMESIS GRAVIDARUM

## Definition

Hyperemesis gravidarum is excessive vomiting during pregnancy.

## Causes

The commonest cause of hyperemesis gravidarum is psychological. A pregnant woman may dislike someone, like her husband, so much that she vomits severely when she sees this person. Other causes of hyperemesis gravidarum include:

- Multiple pregnancy.
- Trophoblastic disease.
- Urinary tract infection.

# Differential diagnosis

A pregnant woman is not immune to suffering from other conditions that can mimic hyperemesis gravidarum.
- Medical conditions like urinary tract infection, pyelonephritis, respiratory tract infection and malaria.
- Surgical conditions like intestinal obstruction and appendicitis.

# Complications

Due to excessive vomiting there is:
- Loss of body fluids leading to dehydration.
- Loss of electrolytes leading to electrolyte imbalance like hypocalcaemia and hypokalaemia.
- Jaundice can occur in severe states and cause liver damage.

# Investigations

The investigations that a ca be performed in a health centre include:
- Urine for microscopy (pus cells, red blood cells, sugar, proteins and acetone).
- Blood slide for malaria parasites.
- In big centres other investigations can be done like urine for culture and sensitivity, blood urea, creatinine, serum electrolytes and ketone bodies in urine.
- Other investigations will depend on the suspected cause.
- In severe states liver function test should be performed.

# Treatment

All patients with hyperemesis gravidarum should be admitted and resuscitated quickly. In resuscitating the patient the author prescribes as follows:
- The patient should take nothing per oral for at least 24 hours.

- Intravenous infusion of 5% Dextrose alternating with Normal Saline or Ringer's lactate, three litres in 24 hours.
- Promethazine injection 50 mg 8 hourly for 24 hours. Other drugs like gravol and chlorpheniramine can be given.

Many of the patients improve within twenty-four hours. When the patient has improved she should be encouraged to drink fluids like tea or fresh orange juice. The patient should also be advised to take small quantities of non-fatty foods, frequently.

Specific treatment depending on the suspected cause is also given. If the condition does not improve within 24 hours such patients should be referred to hospital. In intractable hyperemesis gravidarum, especially if jaundice has developed, the pregnancy may have to be terminated.

# HEARTBURN

Heartburn is common during the last three months of pregnancy. The patient experiences heat under the sternum. Heartburn is due to reflux of gastric secretions into the oesophagus due to relaxation of cardiac sphincter.

## Treatment

- Anti-acids like fresh milk, or mist magnesium trisilicate should be given frequently.
- Hypnotics. If the patient misses sleep sedatives like diazepam can be given in the night.

# CONSTIPATION

It is usual for pregnant women to have constipation. The constipation is due to reduced intestinal peristalsis caused by high levels of progesterone.

In disturbing constipation of like 3–5 days the patient should be advised to take lots of roughage like cabbages or ripe papaw. Laxatives/purgatives during pregnancy are dangerous as they can cause abortion, preterm labour or even dehydration.

# BACKACHE

Low backache is common during pregnancy. The causes of low back-ache are:
- Relaxin, which is a hormone produced by the pregnant woman, relaxes all her body ligaments.
- The increased body weight.
- The lordosis state of the backbone.

Low backache is worse during late pregnancy, especially if the woman has sedentary duties. The treatment of low backache of pregnancy is mainly bed rest.

# ABDOMINAL CRAMPS

Mild abdominal cramps are common especially in late pregnancy. The abdominal cramps could be due to:
- Braxton-Hicks contractions of the uterus.
- Tension of the round ligaments. The round ligaments are stretched as the uterus grows.

The treatment for the abdominal cramps is mainly bed rest.

A PREGNANT WOMAN SHOULD BE ADVISED TO REST BOTH PHYSICAL AND MENTALLY.

# CHAPTER 6

# GYNAECOLOGICAL/OBSTETRICAL HISTORY TAKING AND EXAMINATION

## INTRODUCTION

History taking is the first step and most important in the diagnosis of a disease. A clinician should not rush to examine and /or carry out an investigation on a patient before taking a full and detailed history. Some gynaecological/obstetrical conditions can be diagnosed by history alone and have very few physical signs like dysfunctional uterine bleeding. The principles of gynaecological/ obstetrical history taking, examination and investigation are the same as in other clinical specialties. In other disciplines emphasis is not on the genital organs and thus misdiagnosis and delay in proper management is common; like a pregnant woman who had fallen from a tree and comes to hospital with a broken leg. If proper history is not taken this woman will only get treatment for her leg and the intactness of the pregnancy will be overlooked.

TAKE A THOROUGH GYNAECOLOGICAL/OBSTETRICAL HISTORY IN A WOMAN WHATEVER SHE IS SUFERRING FROM.

History taking and examination is an art, which needs to be practiced frequently for mastery.

# OBJECTIVES

It is expected that the student will be able to:
- List the headlines of a good obstetrical/gynaecological history.
- Take a good gynaecological/obstetrical history.
- Examine a gynaecological/obstetrical patient.
- Perform vaginal examination.

# HEADLINES OF A GOOD GYNAECOLOGI-CAL/OBSTETRICAL HISTORY

A gynaecological/obstetrical history has the following headlines:

## Personal data

Personal data is also known as introduction. In this it is important to include the name, age (either as known by the patient or estimated from a known common event, or onset of menarche or peer person), marital status (married, single, common law relationship, widowed or divorced), occupation and education.

If a patient is pregnant it is helpful to include her gravidity and parity.

## Main complaints

The patient should be asked her problems, which forced her to come to clinic. The list of her complaints is then re-arranged in order of occurrence. Medical diagnoses like anaemia, high blood pressure are not complaints.

## Amplification of complaints

The patient should be asked the state and characteristic of her health before the onset of the complaint. Each complain should then be considered in detail like if the complaint is pain in the lower abdomen the patient should be asked for the location, onset (acute or gradual), intensity, character and radiation. Each symptom can be due to involvement of one or more systems; like abdominal pain can be due to problems in gastrointestinal tract, genital urinary system and even respiratory tract, so other symptoms associated with each system should be asked for.

## Review of other systems

A patient, whether medically trained or not, tends to consider some of her medical problems not contributing to her gynaecological/obstetrical problems. It is therefore important to review all the other systems not complained of. If any significant complaint is discovered this should be included in the list of main complaints and amplified as said earlier. So in the review of systems nothing significant should be complained of.

## Past medical and surgical history

The patient should be asked what diseases she suffered from in the past and the treatment she had. She should also be asked about any surgical interventions including the date and outcome.

If no significant past medical and surgical history, the patient should still be asked for any past history of tuberculosis, heart disease and diabetes mellitus.

## Past gynaecological history

Past gynaecological history is essentially menstrual history. The patient should be asked when she had her menarche and at what age. The average length of her menstrual cycle, the number of days she menstruates and the amount of blood loss in terms of the number of maternity pads she uses per day. Heavy periods are usually accompanied with clots. The patient should be asked if her periods are painful or not. If the periods are painful the character of the pain should be established.

The patient should be asked when she had her LMP, which is the day she started getting her normal menstruation. If the patient is bleeding at the time of the visit this should not be considered to be the normal period but ask her previous period was. Her present bleeding might be abnormal unless she completes it normally.

In a patient who is pregnant the EDD should be calculated and gestation period by date from LMP. A gestational calculator can also be used to determine the EDD and gestational age of the pregnancy.

## Family and social history

There are familial, contagious and hereditary diseases and some social factors, which cause certain diseases, thus, the importance of family and social history.

The health status of the patient's parents and siblings should be known. If a member of her family is ill the type of illness should be explored. If any was dead, the cause of death should be inquired. If the whole family is healthy, still the presence of tuberculosis, heart disease and diabetes mellitus should be excluded. In pregnant patients history of multiple pregnancies should be asked for.

In social history, dietary history and living conditions should be included. In dietary history her usual menu should be ask for instead of allowing her to list the types of food, as some tend to exaggerate.

## Past obstetrical history

If the patient is pregnant her gravidity included otherwise her parity is the only one noted. For each pregnancy it is important to include the year, at what gestation period she delivered (if it was not full term the reason of preterm delivery or abortion should be noted and whether the uterus was evacuated). The mode of delivery; if abnormal like delivery by caesarean section, the reason and outcome should be asked for. The sex of the baby, its weight and health status are important. Any complications during pregnancy, labour and puerperium and how she was managed should be noted.

## Other minor headlines

Other minor headlines will depend on the type of patient:
   • History of sexual relationships. This is more important in the infertile couple. The frequency of coitus per week and whether she feels pains or not should be asked for.
   • History of contraceptives is important for all patients. The type of contraceptives and when it was stopped is important.

## Summary of history

It is advisable to summarize the history especially during examination times. When making a summary the positive and important negative findings leading to a certain diagnosis are included.

> TAKE A DETAILED HISTORY. DO NOT LEAVE A
> STONE UNTURNED.

# PHYSICAL EXAMINATION

Note that women are shy of having their bodies examined. The examiner should always be gentle and nice to the patient. The patient should give a verbal consent for the examination. Patients should not be over-expose.

The examination should be done in a private room in the presence of a female nurse especially if the examiner is a male.

Examination of the patient starts from the time she enters into the clinic. The patient should be examined from head to toe and not only the abdomen and pelvic organs.

> **A WOMAN IS A TOTAL HUMAN-BEING AND NOT ONLY MADE OF THE ABDOMEN AND PELVIC ORGANS.**

The examination starts with inspection then palpation, percussion and lastly auscultation. The patient should lie on a comfortable examination couch where there is good illumination, preferably sunlight. The patient should have her legs straight and lie flat or with one pillow under her head unless she has orthopnoea (breathlessness on lying flat). The findings can be grouped as such:

- General examination. As described under the chapter on Antenatal care.
- Systemic examination. As said under the chapter on antenatal care.
- Abdominal Examination.
  The general examination is as said under the antenatal care. Before palpation the patient should be asked to show where she feels pain on her abdomen. The palpation should start away from the painful site and work clockwise or anti-clockwise. It is advisable to start with superficial palpation so as to get the areas

with obvious tenderness and enlarged masses. Deep palpation is for identifying any enlarged masses especially the spleen, liver and kidneys. Any palpable mass should be described in terms of its site, size, consistency, tenderness, mobility and whether the mass is under the muscles, in the muscles or under the skin. Rebound tenderness should be checked if peritonitis is suspected. Fluid thrill and shifting dullness should be elicited if ascites is suspicion.

➤ Percussion of the abdomen for dullness or resonance.
➤ Auscultation of the abdomen for bowel movements.

If the patient is pregnant she should be examined as described under the chapter on antenatal care.

• Vaginal examination.

Vaginal examination is very important, but unfortunately this examination involves the private parts of the patient. Unless the examiner has a good rapport with the patient and the patient has confidence in him/her she may resist this examination.

---

**THE PATIENT SHOULD BE ASSURED CONFIDENTIALITY OF HER FINDINGS.**

---

The patient should have her bladder emptied before the examination. The patient should remove her underwear, flex her legs and abduct them and relax. The patient should be assured that the examination is not painful as it will be done gently.

➤ Inspection of the vulva for obvious discharges, swellings, sores, or any local inflammation. The hymen should also be examined. The urethral meatus should be inspected for discharge and inflammation.
➤ Speculum examination is done using Cusco's (bivalve) speculum to view the cervix. If the vaginal wall needs to be visualized

the patient is put into Sim's position (the patient lies on her left lateral position, extends her left leg while the right leg is flexed) and Sim's speculum used.

➢ Bimanual examination of the pelvic organs is done next.

VAGINAL EXAMINATION NEEDS SKILLS ONLY LEARNT BY FREQUENT PRACTICE UNDER SUPERVISION OF A SKILLED OBSTETRICIAN/ /MIDWIFE.

- Rectal examination. Rectal examination can be done in virgins where bimanual pelvic examination is not advisable. By performing rectal examination the ovaries, tubes and uterus can be palpated.

# CHAPTER 7

# ANTENATAL CARE (A.N.C)

## INTRODUCTION

Good antenatal care of a pregnant woman will assure her delivery of a healthy baby and her own health too. A woman who had no good antenatal care stands a high chance of losing her baby and/or her own life. Good antenatal care lowers maternal and perinatal mortality rates.

## OBJECTIVES

The student should be able to:
- Define antenatal care.
- List the objectives of antenatal care.
- Organize an antenatal clinic.
- Take a good obstetric history.
- Examine a pregnant mother in particular the pregnant uterus.
- Detect a "high risk" pregnant woman.

## DEFINITION

Antenatal care is the care given to a pregnant woman.

# OBJECTIVES OF ANTENATAL CARE

The overall objective of antenatal care is to ensure that the pregnant woman reaches the end of her pregnancy healthy, physically and mentally, and at the end delivers a live and healthy baby. Many complications during pregnancy and delivery can be predicted, diagnosed and prevented during the antenatal period.

To be able to attain the main objective the following specific objectives relate to antenatal care:
- To ensure a good standard of health to all pregnant women.
- To select those women who might encounter a problem (high risk) in pregnancy or labour and take the necessary steps early.
- To observe any abnormality in the pregnancy and advise the woman the best course of action thereafter.
- To deal with any common illnesses during pregnancy.
- To make the mother aware of the benefits offered by antenatal, postnatal and family planning clinics.

# FUNCTIONS OF ANTENATAL CLINIC

To be able to attain the main objective of A.N.C. the following are done at clinic:
- Examine pregnant women.
- Treat minor ailments of pregnancy.
- Immunize pregnant women against tetanus.
- Give prophylaxis against malaria and anaemia.
- Refer the high-risk women to hospital.
- Give health education to pregnant women.
- Counsel and provide family planning methods.

# The flow of patients in MCH/FP clinics

To prevent patients from colliding with one another the one way flow of patients is recommended as the sketch below shows:

- Station A can be outside the MCH/FP building (at the veranda). Medically non-trained personnel who knows how to read and write is enough. In this station recording of laboratory results and other investigations, as urine for protein and haemoglobin estimation using the talquist method can be done here. The weight and height of pregnant women and children are also done here.
- Station $B_1$ & $B_2$ should be inside the MCH/FP building. The rooms need to be adequate, comfortable and have enough privacy. Trained personnel like MCH/FP aides could be stationed here. In station $B_2$ patients' history taking, examination and counselling for family planning are done. It is also advisable to supply contraceptives at station $B_2$, confidentially.
- Station C can be in a small room within the building. A medically untrained person who knows how to read and write can manage station C. In this station dispensing of drugs like iron, folic acid and chloroquine is done together with immunization of both the children and mothers.

# One-way patient flow diagram

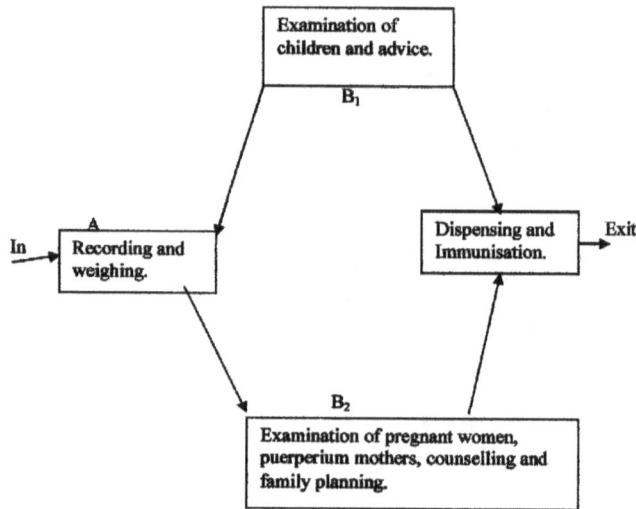

One-way patient flow diagram

# THE FIRST ANTENATAL VISIT

The activities carried out during the first antenatal visit include:
- Registration.
- Weight and height measurement.
- History taking.
- Physical examination.
- Laboratory investigations.
- Management of minor complaints.
- Prophylactic treatment.

- Immunization.
- Health education.

## Registration

All pregnant women should be registered and given an antenatal card (see appendix–1).

## Weight and height measurement

The weight can be measured using a bathroom scale. The woman should have as few clothes as possible. The weighing scale should be checked frequently for accuracy. The weight is taken in kilograms. The height is taken in centimetres by asking the woman to stand bare footed against a graduated wall. If there is a weighing machine which has length scale the height of the patient can be taken simultaneously with her weight.

## History taking

History taking is done in station $B_2$ of the flow pattern. The history should be as described in chapter–6.

## Physical examination

Physical examination should be exhaustive. This might be the first and/or last time the woman visits a health institution. The woman should thus be examined thoroughly.

- General examination of the patient starts from the time she comes into the antenatal clinic which include:
  Patient's general outlook, whether ill-looking or not.
  - ➢ Nutritional status. Signs of wasting include prominent zygomatic bones, wasted intercostal spaces, and hypothenar and thenar muscles.

➤ Blood pressure estimation. This is taken at station A while the patient is seated. If the blood pressure is noted to be high it should be repeated while the patient is lying laterally. Taking the blood pressure when the patient is in a dorsal position can lower the blood pressure or even cause hypotension (Supine Hypotensive Syndrome). This lowering of blood pressure is due to the gravid uterus compressing the inferior vena cava and/or the abdominal aorta.

➤ Pallor indicates anaemia. This is searched for in the subconjuctiva, tongue, mouth, palms, finger, nails, and soles of feet and even in the vaginal wall.

➤ Examination of the breasts.

• Systemic examination should be done.

➤ Cardiovascular system especially pulse rate, size of heart, heart sounds and murmurs.

➤ Respiratory system to rule out pulmonary tuberculosis and any other lung lesions.

➤ Musculo-skeletal system in particular the pelvis and the spine, to rule out bony abnormalities.

➤ Central nervous system should be examined if indicated.

• Examination of the pregnant abdomen is very important. All the time the examiner should be fast and gentle as the patient gets tired easily.

➤ The patient should lie supine and pull her clothes down to the mons pubis and the chest short of exposing the breasts.

➤ Inspection of the abdomen for distension anteriorly and on the flanks. Inspection of the overlying skin for any marks.

➤ Palpation of fundus of the uterus and estimate its level as described in chapter–4. The fundal height is compared with the gestation period in dates as calculated from L.M.P.

➤ The lie of the foetus is determined. Lie of the foetus is the relationship of the long axis of the foetus to that of the mother.

The lie can be longitudinal (normal), transverse, or oblique. The lie can be determined by palpating the back of the foetus, which feels smooth and regular. The lie of the foetus is most important after 32 weeks of pregnancy. Before 32 weeks of gestation the lie has no significance. Before 32 weeks the uterus is larger than the foetus thus the foetus keeps on changing its lie.

➢ The presentation of the foetus should be determined. Presentation is the leading part of the foetus. The presentation can be either cephalic (head presenting; round, hard and ballotable), breech (buttocks presenting, soft and irregular).

➢ Attitude of the foetal parts is the relationship of the foetal parts to one another. Weight of the foetus should be estimated.

➢ The foetal heart should be searched. The foetal heart is best heard over the area where the foetal spine is and towards its head.

➢ Position of the presentation. This is the relationship of the denominator of the presentation to the maternal pelvis. The position of the foetus can accurately be detected by doing vaginal examination and not by abdominal examination.

## Routine laboratory examination

The following investigations should be done to all women during their first antenatal visit:

• Haemoglobin estimation. This is commonly estimated by using the talquist method, which is cheaper and faster. Every clinic should have one booklet of talquist. If used economically one booklet can be used for up to six months in a clinic which attends 100 women per day. Other instruments for haemoglobin estimation include Lovebond comparator, Shale method and Electro-photometer. Electro-photometer is most reliable.

- Proteinuria is the presence of protein in urine. This can be estimated by using the albustic. Other methods of estimating protein in urine include the boiling method, cold method (Salicylic Sulphonic acid) and the esbach method but these methods are not commonly used. Urine should also be examined for pus cells (pregnant women are more prone to getting urinary tract infection than non-pregnant ones). Schistosoma ova should be looked for in urine in areas where schistosomal infection is possible. The commonest schistosomal ovum in Tanzania is Schistosoma haematobium.
- Stool should be examined for ova especially hookworm and ascaris ova.
- Blood group and Rhesus factor must be determined.
- Test for syphilis (VDRL = Venereal Disease Research Laboratory).
- Test for Human Immune Virus.

## Management of Minor Ailments of Pregnancy

The minor ailments of pregnancy (see chapter–5) complained of by the patient should not be ignored as they can cause discomfort and misery to the woman or even interfere with her nutrition. Try to treat or alleviate the minor ailments.

## Routine prophylaxis

- Malaria is pan-endemic in Tanzania. Mosquitoes are even found in cold highlands like Usambara Mountains. It is thus recommended to give anti-malaria prophylaxis to all pregnant women. Pregnant women should be given chloroquine tablets 300 mg (2 tablets) weekly until end of puerperium. Many women think that chloroquine can cause abortion or preterm labour so they do not take the tablets. This fear should be alleviated and the women encouraged taking the chloroquine. Many midwives do not advise women to continue taking chloroquine after delivery, but this is bad as women succumb to malarial attacks easily during the puerperal period too.

- Anaemia, in particular the iron deficiency type, is very common in the third world, more so, in pregnant women. Give pregnant women iron tablets like ferrous sulphate (200 mg), fumarate (200mg) or succinate (100mg). These drugs can be given once a day if the haemoglobin is 10.0mg/dl or more (if the patient's haemoglobin is 11.0mg/dl or more the author does not give iron tablets but just encourages the patient on diet), twice a day if the haemoglobin is less than 10.0 mg/dl but 9.0 mg/dl or more and thrice a day if the haemoglobin is less than 9 mg/dl. Many women dislike taking the iron tablets for, to some, it causes nausea. A woman who takes iron tablets has black stools. Pregnant women should be encouraged to take the iron tablets. If the patient prefers liquid iron it is okay.
- Folic acid deficiency is also common in pregnant women. All pregnant women should be given folic acid 5mg daily. Folic acid is also known to prevent development of Neural Tubal Defects (NTD) in the foetus so it is recommended to also be taken before conception.
- Calcium tablets. It is now recommended that all pregnant women should be given calcium supplements.

## Immunization of pregnant women

To prevent tetanus neonatorum, which is a great killer of newborn babies in the third world, W.H.O. has produced a new schedule for immunization against tetanus as per appendix–2. This immunization programme should be started for all school attending girls so that by the time they get into reproductive age they are fully immunized against tetanus

## Health education

The midwife should take advantage of the A.N.C. for health education. Group health education can be done at station A of the MCH / FP flow pattern. The midwife should select topics relevant to his/ her target group or try to do community needs assessment so as to get relevant topics.

## Nutrition

The pregnant woman should be advised on the available and affordable food to eat. She should be advised to eat balanced diet. The advice of a nutritionist, if available, should be sort

# RE-ATTENDANCE TO A.N.C

The pregnant woman should be encouraged to re-visit A.N.C. After each visit the woman should be told the date of her next visit and the date written on her antenatal card which she takes home. It is advisable that the re-visits are scheduled to be on the same day of the week for each woman. The clinic should not be delayed or prolonged for doing so will discourage the women from coming back to the clinic. The average schedule for seeing pregnant women is:

- Once per month for the first twenty-eight weeks of pregnancy.
- Once a fortnight from the 28th week to the 36th weeks of pregnancy.
- Once every week from the 36th week of pregnancy to delivery.

Note that patients with no high risk factors can be seen less frequent as suggested above. This will reduce the unnecessary overcrowding of patients in the clinic. Those with high risk factors will get the attention needed.

The activities during the re-visit period are as during the first visit but brief:

> ➤ History taking is merely for any recent problems.
> ➤ Examination is brief. Pallor, blood pressure, weight oedema of ankles should be looked
> ➤ The abdomen should be examined, in particular the uterus as during the first visit.

- Proteinuria should be looked for in every visit.
- Haemoglobin should be estimated monthly. If this is not possible the haemoglobin should be done at least three times in the whole antenatal period; preferably at first visit, at 28 weeks of pregnancy and at 36 weeks of pregnancy.

THE HAEMOGLOBIN OF A PREGNANT WOMAN SHOULD BE CHECKED EVERY MONTH.

During all the visits, the patient should be told about the findings and what they mean. All the questions the woman might should be answered. The necessary action of findings during the woman's visit should be taken. All the findings should be record in the antenatal card.

BEING NICE AND KIND TO A PREGNANT WOMAN ENHANCES RAPPORT.

# THE HIGH RISK FACTORS

During the first and subsequent visits the midwife should try to rule out any high risk factor(s) and take the necessary line of action as shown in the antenatal card (see appendix–1). All patients found to have high risk factors should be referred to hospital early enough for delivery. If the clinic is near a hospital all such patients should attend the hospital's clinic, otherwise they can be managed at the health centre and be transferred to hospital for delivery at 38 weeks of gestation. The factors, which put a woman in high-risk group, include:

- Past obstetric history:
  - ➢ Previous operative deliveries like caesarean section, vacuum extraction, symphysiotomy, laparotomy for ruptured uterus and forceps deliveries.
  - ➢ Retained placenta.
  - ➢ Postpartum haemorrhage.
  - ➢ Three or more consecutive spontaneous abortions.
  - ➢ Previous stillbirths or neonatal deaths.
  - ➢ Grand multiparity (4+).
  - ➢ History of 10+ years of involuntary infertility.
- Past gynaecological operations:
  - ➢ Repaired vaginal fistulae.
  - ➢ Repaired genital prolapse.
  - ➢ Repaired third degree perineal tear.
- Primigravida:
  - ➢ Height 145 cm or less (short primigravida).
  - ➢ Age 35 years and above (elderly primigravida) or below 16 years (young primigravida).
  - ➢ Teenager that is age below 20 years.
  - ➢ Deformities of musculo-skeletal system, like kyphosis, deformed pelvis or legs due to polio, tuberculosis, injury.
- Maternal diseases:
  - ➢ PIH (Pregnancy Induced Hypertension).
  - ➢ Blood pressure of 130/90 mm Hg and above or increase of diastolic blood pressure of 15 mm Hg or systolic pressure of 30 mm Hg above the pre-pregnant blood pressure.
  - ➢ Haemoglobin level of (8 g/dl) or less.
  - ➢ Diseases of the heart, lungs and kidneys; diabetes mellitus and syphilis.

➢ Uterine fibroid and other pelvic masses or abdominal tumors.

➢ STI especially HIV and syphilis.

- Abnormal pregnancy:
  ➢ Multiple pregnancy.
  ➢ Malpresentation of the foetus.
  ➢ Abnormal lie of the foetus.
  ➢ Intra-uterine foetal death.
  ➢ Polyhydramnios.
  ➢ A.P.H. (Antepartum Haemorrhage).
  ➢ Intra-uterine foetal growth retardation.
- Complications arising during labour.
  ➢ Foetal distress.
  ➢ Prolonged labour.
  ➢ Premature rupture of membranes.
  ➢ Preterm labour.
  ➢ Hyperpyrexia.
  ➢ Intrauterine foetal death.
- At the end of every visit tell the when she is expected to deliver, how she will probably deliver and when she should go to hospital for the delivery; so that she prepares herself ahead of time.

THE IDENTIFIED HIGH RISK FACTOR SHOULD BE WRITTEN ON TOP OF THE ANTENATAL CARD IN RED INK BEFORE THE PATIENT IS REFERRED.

# CHAPTER 8

# MALPRESENTATION AND ABNORMAL LIE

## INTRODUCTION

Over 90% of singleton babies lie longitudinally and present by the vertex. Any foetal lie other than longitudinal or presentation other than vertex is abnormal. Malpresentation and/or abnormal lie are accompanied by abnormal labour. Labour in malpresentation and abnormal lie may either be prolonged or need operative delivery. Recognition of malpresentation or abnormal lie during the antenatal period or early in labour is very paramount. Malpresentation includes cord presentation/prolapse, face, brow, shoulder and breech. Abnormal lie includes transverse, oblique and unstable lie.

## OBJECTIVES

The student is expected to be able to:
- Define presentation and lie of foetus.
- Diagnose malpresentation and abnormal lie.
- Manage malpresentation and abnormal lie before transfer.
- Assist breech delivery.

# DEFINITIONS

- Presentation is defined as the leading part of the foetus or that part of the foetus near to the pelvic brim.
- Lie is defined as the relationship of the long axis of the foetus to the maternal spine or the relationship of the foetal spine to the long axis of the uterus.

# CORD PROLAPSE

Cord prolapse occurs when the umbilical cord passes into the vagina ahead of the presenting part. The cord may lie enclosed in the intact bag of fore-waters, often called cord presentation, or may have prolapsed into the vagina after rupture of amniotic membrane, this is called cord prolapse.

## Causes or cord prolapse/presentation

Any condition where the presenting part of the foetus does not fit well into the pelvis will favour prolapse/presentation of the cord. Some of the conditions include:

- Cephalo-pelvic disproportion due to contracted pelvis, big baby or hydrocephalus.
- Malpresentation of the foetus e.g. breech, shoulder presentation.
- Abnormal lie of the foetus like transverse and oblique lie.
- Multiple pregnancy.
- Polyhydramnios.
- Rupture of membranes before the head is engaged.

## Management of cord prolapse or presentation

If the membranes are intact and the cord is presenting the cord could be pushed back. For cord prolapse the management depends on the condition of the foetus (maturity and lie) and the degree of cervical dilatation.

- If the cord is not pulsating, indicating foetal death, foetal delivery in the health centre can be done unless there is contracted pelvis or any other malpresentation and/or abnormal lie.
- If the cord is pulsating (indicating that the foetus is alive) and the foetus is sufficiently mature to live outside the uterus, then management of such a patient depends on the cervical dilatation.

If the cervix is fully dilated, then delivery should be done immediately. If the presenting part is vertex, vacuum extraction should be performed immediately. If the presenting part is breech, then breech extraction should be done immediately.

If the cervix is not fully dilated the cord is packed into the vagina immediately. The patient should be put in Knee-chest position or Trendelenburg's position or modified Sim's position. A hand is pushed into the vagina so as to push the presenting part upward to prevent or minimize cord compression. The patient is referred to hospital in any of the above positions. While transferring the patient the hand in the vagina should continue to push the presenting part upwards.

## Prognosis in cord prolapse

Cord prolapse is an emergency condition accompanied by high perinatal mortality (20–60 %).

## Prevention of cord prolapse

- Artificial rupture of membranes should not be done when the foetal head is high, breech presentation, transverse lie, oblique lie or in multiple pregnancy.
- In cord presentations, when membranes are intact, push back the cord before rupturing the membranes.
- During artificial rupture of membranes the liquor should not be released fast.

> CORD PROLAPSE SHOULD BE RULED OUT WHENEVER MEMBRANES RUPTURE.

# FACE PRESENTATION

The diagnosis of face presentation is correctly done on vaginal examination. In face presentation the orbital ridges of eyes will feel (care should be taken not to damage the eyes) and the irregular nose and mouth. When much oedema has occurred face presentation may be mistaken for breech. To differentiate breech the anus of the foetus may grip the examining finger whereas the mouth will not do so. After delivery the foetus, which was presenting by face, its lips will be distorted and oedematous.

## Causes of face presentation

Mostly, the cause of face presentation is not known. At times face presentation is due to foetal abnormalities like anencephaly, tumor of foetal neck and shortening of the foetal neck muscles, or brow presentation which turns to face presentation during labour.

## Management of face presentation

Management of face presentation depends on the position of the mentum which is its denominator.

- In mento-anterior position the presenting diameter is the sub-mento-bregmatic (9.5cm). Majority of such foetuses can be delivered vaginally.
- In mento-posterior the presenting diameter is the sterno-bregmatic (18cm). Such a baby can not be delivered vaginally. Such patients should be referred to hospital for emergency caesarean section.

# BROW PRESENTATION

Brow presentation can mostly be diagnosed by vaginal examination. The palpation of the anterior fontanelle and the supra-orbital ridges indicates brow presentation.

## Management of Brow Presentation

Brow presentation is the most unfavourable of all the cranial presentations of the foetus. In brow presentation the mento-vertical diameter (14.0cm) presents and this will not pass through the pelvic inlet. When brow presentation is diagnosed during labour the delivery is by caesarean section, thus such a woman should be referred to hospital immediately.

# SHOULDER PRESENTATION

In shoulder presentation the baby is either in transverse or oblique lie.

## Cause of oblique/transverse lie

The cause of transverse or oblique lie may be unknown but this lie is common in:
- Large uterus, as in multigravida and polyhydramnios, as the baby can assume any lie comfortably.
- Multiple pregnancy, as the foetuses can splint one another, thus preventing one from lying longitudinally.
- Placenta praevia, as there is not enough space in the pelvis.

# SHOULDER PRESENTATION

In shoulder presentation the baby is either in transverse or oblique lie.

## Cause of oblique/transverse lie

The cause of transverse or oblique lie may be unknown but this lie is common in:
- Large uterus, as in multigravida and polyhydramnios, as the baby can assume any lie comfortably.
- Multiple pregnancy, as the foetuses can splint one another, thus preventing one from lying longitudinally.
- Placenta praevia, as there is not enough space in the pelvis.
- Congenital malformations of the uterus like arcuate and septate uterus.
- Contracted pelvis.

## Diagnosis of transverse/oblique lie

- In transverse lie.
  - ➢ The abdomen is enlarged transversely and is transverse oval.
  - ➢ The flanks of the abdomen are enlarged.
  - ➢ The fundal height is is smaller than dates.

> There is no foetal head felt in the pelvis or fundus of the uterus. The foetal head might be felt on the sides of the abdomen.
> The foetus lies crosswise or obliqually.

- In oblique lie.
  > The abdomen looks normal and the fundal height correlates with the gestational age
  > The presenting part is found on either the left or right iliac fossa regions not in the lower pole of the uterus.
  > On vaginal examination a foetal hand, arm, elbow or tip of the shoulder may be felt in the pelvis. The hand defers from the heel in that the hand can be straightened out at the wrist and no palpable calcaneus bone. The thumb of a hand is shorter then the rest of the fingers while toes are approximately of the same length.

## Management of transverse/oblique lie

If oblique/transverse lie is diagnosed in a health centre the patient should be referred to hospital after 32 weeks of pregnancy for possible external cephalic version (ECV).

| THE DIAGNOSIS OF TRANSVERSE/OBLIQUE LIE BEFORE 32 WEEKS OF GESTATION HAS NO SIGNIFICANCE. |
| --- |

If ECV fails or is contra-indicated, the delivery of the baby is by caesarean section.

| ARM/HAND PROLAPSE IS COMMON IN TRANSVERSE/OBLIQUE LIE. |
| --- |

# UNSTABLE LIE

In unstable lie the foetus is found to be in a different lie each time. Unstable lie can be diagnosed after 32 weeks gestation and not before. Before 32 weeks of gestation the foetus can assume any lie without being abnormal. Unstable lie is commonly found in multigravida of high parity and polyhydramnios. If the health centre is near a hospital, patients with unstable lie should attend the antenatal clinic of the hospital for correction of any abnormal lie. If the health centre is far from hospital and the patient has no relatives near the hospital, she could be managed at the health centre and referred to the hospital after 37 completed weeks.

In hospital she will be watched and any abnormal lie corrected. She is allowed to go into labour and frequently the uterine muscles straighten out the lie of the foetus. If the lie is oblique or transverse before labour starts ECV can be done and rupture of membranes performed.

# BREECH PRESENTATION

In breech presentation the foetus presents with buttocks. Breech presentation is common (4% of all presentations). In early pregnancy breech presentation is common. At 20 weeks about 15%, and at 34 weeks about 6% of foetuses present as breech. By the 34th week of gestation over three-quarters of breech presentations have undergone spontaneous cephalic version.

## Causes of breech presentation

The causes of persistent breech after 34 weeks are mostly unknown. Other causes of breech presentation include:
- Contracted pelvis.

- Placenta praevia
- Abnormal uterus like septate uterus or myoma of uterus.
- Abnormal attitude of foetus (deflexed head and extended legs).

## Types of breech presentation

There are three types of breech:
- Extended breech also known as "Frank breech". In this type of breech both of the foetus's legs lie along its abdomen and splint its body.
- Flexed breech, also known as "Complete breech". In this type of breech the legs are flexed together and the breech sits with the flexed legs.
- Footling breech. Usually in this type of breech one leg is flexed while the other is straightened downwards. In this type of breech prolapse of the foot is possible before delivery of the breech.

## Diagnosis of breech presentation

It is important that the diagnosis of breech presentation is made before 36 weeks of pregnancy so that version can be attempted. As said earlier, diagnosing breech before 32 weeks of gestation should not raise any anxiety as by the 34th week of gestation only a quarter of the breech presentation will persist to be so.

The diagnosis of breech is mainly by physical examination-and investigation. Sometimes the patient may admit that she feels the baby kicking in the lower abdomen, but this is an unreliable symptom.
- On palpation of the uterus the fundus will be found to be occupied by a firm, smooth, round and ballottable mass which indicates the head. The breech can be well felt by the "Pawlick's" grip rather than the ordinary bimanual one.

- The foetal heart may be heard clearly above the umbilicus. In Frank breech and when the buttocks are engaged in the pelvis, the foetal heart may be heard below the umbilicus. Thus the sign of foetal heart is equivocal.
- Vaginal examination, done at the proper time, will reveal a soft and irregular mass instead of a smooth and round mass with palpable sutures indicating the head.
- X-ray of the abdomen is recommended after the 36th week of pregnancy. The aim of the X-ray is to confirm the diagnosis, determine foetal maturity and attitude of the foetus and for pelvimetry.
- In centres where ultra-sound machine is available X-raying should be abandoned in favour of the ultrasound.

## Dangers of breech presentation

Maternal risks in breech presentation are slightly greater than in vertex presentation since breech delivery frequently needs operative intervention.

Foetal risks in breech delivery are high unless an elective caesarean section if performed in time. In assisted breech delivery the foetal risks depend on:

- The skill of the midwife and his/her team. The more experienced the midwife is the lower the risk.
- Weight of the baby. If the baby weighs less than 2.250 kgs, the foetal mortality is 12% (prematurity is the main cause of death). If the baby's weight is between 2.250 kgs and 3.500 kgs the mortality is 5%. If the foetal weight is greater than 3.500 kgs the mortality rate is 10% due to high chances of the foetal head or shoulders getting stuck.

The principal causes of foetal mortality of babies weighing more 3.500 kgs are:
- Asphyxia from prolapse cord. This accident can occur in even lighter babies.
- Intra-cranial haemorrhage due to tentorial tears; from traumatic vaginal delivery.
- Fractures of femur, humerus or clavicle may occur during delivery.
- Head and/or shoulder arrest.

## Management of breech presentation

During pregnancy refer all diagnosed breech presentation to hospital for external cephalic version unless the version is contraindicated. The patients should be referred to hospital between 32 and 36 weeks of pregnancy. Version before 32 weeks of pregnancy is pointless and version after 36 weeks of pregnancy is difficult to perform. Version is contraindicated in-patients with:
- Previous history of caesarean section, for fear of tearing the scar.
- Placenta praevia for fear of causing bleeding.
- Multiple pregnancy, as this is difficult, due to the other foetus.
- PIH for fear of abruptio placenta.
- Elderly primigravida for fear of the complications of version which include onset of preterm labour, premature rupture of membranes, abruptio placenta and knotting of cord.

ECV SHOULD NOT BE DONE BY A CLINICAL OFFICER/MIDWIFE.

# The mode of delivering a breech

- Caesarean section should be done in patients with suspected contracted pelvis, primigravida, patients with other high risk factors or if second stage of labour is delayed.

PROLONGED/DELAYED SECOND STAGE OF LABOUR IN BREECH PRESENTATION MAY MEAN DISPROPORTION.

- Vaginal delivery of a breech increases the risks of the foetus more than caesarean section (see dangers of breech presentation). A Clinical Officer/midwife is not supposed to assist breech delivery in a health centre. Selection of patients for vaginal delivery and the assisting of the delivery need special skills. There are times when a Clinical Officer/midwife is forced to assist the delivery of a breech either because the mother came in late first stage or is already in second stage of labour. The vaginal delivery of a breech can be by breech extraction that is, pulling down the baby through the pelvis with little or no maternal effort). Breech extraction is rarely done except in the delivery of second twin. The commonest and recommended method of vaginal breech delivery is the "Assisted Breech Delivery".

The first stage of breech delivery is managed as for normal delivery.

PROLONGED FIRST STAGE IS A BAD SIGN.

There should not be any contraindication to vaginal delivery. The presentation and adequacy of the pelvis should be confirmed.

NO TRIAL OF LABOUR IN BREECH PRESENTATION.

If the membranes are ruptured cord prolapse should be ruled out.

> **DO NOT RUPTURE MEMBRANES IN BREECH PRESENTATION.**

The second stage of labour is not prolonged, as is generally believed. Prolonged second stage may mean disproportion.

When the woman is in second stage she should be put in lithotomy position with buttocks to the end of the bed. The woman should not bear down until the foetal buttocks are seen distending the perineum. The woman is then encouraged to bear down with each uterine contraction. As the breech makes its characteristic climb up the perineum, an episiotomy is done. The episiotomy helps to eliminate obstruction at the perineum and also decreases the pressure of the perineum on the head during, head delivery.

The presenting part should not be pulled down until the baby's trunk is born to the level of the umbilicus. Unnecessary interference with the process of breech delivery can cause problems (either shoulders or head will be stuck).

> **DO NOT FORCE VAGINAL BREECH DELIVERY.**

As the umbilicus is born the cord is pulled down gently so as to prevent cord compression. The cord may tear if pulled roughly. After the climb up movement, the foetus flops down. The ventral side of the baby should not be allowed to face upwards at this stage. With further bearing down efforts of the mother, the baby will be born to its neck. When the hair-line of the baby's head appears then the head should be delivered within 10 minutes; but at least 5 minutes should be allowed for the head to descend further. The woman should stop bearing down and the midwife now assists the delivery of the head.

The modern method of assisting the delivery of the head is the Burns-Marshall technique, fig.–13. In this technique the baby is allowed to hang by its own weight from the vulva. As the hairs of the nape of the child's head are seen, both legs of the baby are held and a firm outward force exerted. The baby is drawn over the maternal pubis. This movement will deliver the baby's head. The perineum should be guarded so that the head is delivered slowly.

Burns-Marshall technique can be repeated once or more times if the head is not delivered. Sometimes an assistant may be needed to assist the delivered of the head by pushing the baby's head downwards, abdominally. As the mouth and nose of the baby are born mucus suction is started to clear the baby's airway.

An alternative method of assisting the delivery of the head is the Maurice-Smelli-Veit manoeuvre. The middle finger of a fully pronated left hand is placed on the baby's sub-ccipital region, the ring and index fingers are placed over the shoulders. A supinated right hand is placed below the baby lying astride the arm. One finger of the right hand is placed into the mouth of the foetus and one finger on each molar bone. Pushing the foetal head at the occiput using the right hand and flexion effects delivery of the baby and delivery of the head is done by the left hand by pulling the baby following the curve of the sacrum. Also in this method an assistant can help delivery of the head by pushing the head abdominally.

> MANY TIMES A DIFFICULT BREECH ASSISTED AT A HEALTH CENTRE ENDS UP WITH A DEAD BABY. THEREFORE A CLINICAL OFFICER/MIDWIFE SHOULD NOT BE OVER-CONFIDENT.

> IT IS SAFER TO PERFORM AN ELECTIVE CAESAREAN SECTION THEN TRYING ASSISTED BREECH DELIVERY.

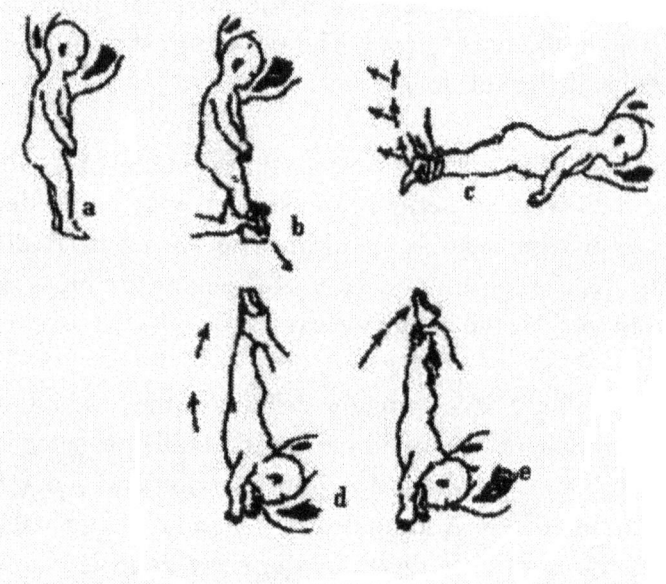

Fig. 13  Burns-Marshall technique

# CHAPTER 9

# MULTIPLE PREGNANCY

## INTRODUCTION

Multiple pregnancies are common worldwide. In Muhimbili Hospital, Tanzania, Dr. Mgaya found that multiple pregnancies occurs 1: 64 pregnancies. Multiple pregnancies, especially twins, occur more frequently in Africans and Asians than in Caucasians and least in Mongolian race. Though a Clinical Officer is expected to refer patients with multiple pregnancy to hospital many a time he/she is forced to assist the delivery of these patients, thus the importance of knowing about multiple pregnancy.

## OBJECTIVES

The student is expected to be able to:
- Define multiple pregnancy.
- Diagnose multiple pregnancy.
- Differentiate between binovular and uniovular twins.
- List the complications of multiple pregnancy.
- Manage a patient with multiple pregnancy during the antenatal period.
- Conduct a delivery of a patient with multiple pregnancy.
- Prevent retention of second twin and management of a retained twin.

# DEFINITION

Multiple pregnancy means that there is more than one foetus present in the uterus. The commonest type of multiple pregnancy is twins.

# CAUSES OF MULTIPLE PREGNANCY

Mostly the cause of multiple pregnancy is not known. Some suspected causes included:
- Familial tendency. Multiple pregnancy is more common in women with familial history of multiple pregnancy.
- Age of the patient. More common in the old pregnant women.
- High parity. More common in the high parous women.
- Injudicious use of fertility drugs, such as clomiphene, during the treatment of infertility.

# DIAGNOSIS OF MULTIPLE PREGNANCY

Multiple pregnancy can be diagnosed during pregnancy by history, examination and investigations. It is not rare to have undiagnosed multiple pregnancy and the woman is found to deliver more than one foetus.

## Symptoms suggestive of Multiple Pregnancy
- During history taking, at antenatal clinic those who have the above factors of causes of multiple pregnancy should be considered to have high chances of having multiple pregnancy. A woman, who has had a multiple pregnancy in her previous pregnancy, is likely to have multiple pregnancy in the present pregnancy.
- The woman may complain of excessive symptoms of pregnancy as compared with her previous pregnancies.

- The patient might admit that she feels too heavy for the gestation period of her pregnancies.
- She may complain of feeling too tired as compared with previous pregnancies.

## Signs suggestive of Multiple Pregnancy

- The woman might have excessive signs of pregnancy like salivation, nausea and vomiting.
- Her abdomen might look pendulous.
- The uterus feels bigger than dates.
- Feeling many foetal parts in the uterus.
- Palpating more than two foetal poles.
- The sign of auscultating two foetal hearts is unreliable. For it to make any meaning two examiners should be listening for the foetal heart at different and opposite points; the foetal heart sounds should be of the same intensity and the heart rate should differ at least by 10 beats per minute.

## Investigation for Multiple Pregnancy

The investigation should be done only if there is a high suspicion index of multiple pregnancy.

- A Clinical Officer can order abdominal X-ray where facilities are available. Note that X-rays could be dangerous to the gonads of both the foetus and mother, thus the X-ray should be taken once and at a gestation period when it is more useful. The aims of taking the X-ray are to determine the number, lie and maturity of the foetuses' and rule out any skeletal congenital malformations.
- If there is a centre with an ultra-sound machine it is advisable to refer all such patients to this centre instead of X-raying. By use of

ultrasound multiple pregnancy can be diagnosed as early as seven weeks of pregnancy.

# TWIN PREGNANCIES

Twin pregnancies are more common than triplets or quadruplets. The twin babies can either be binovular or uniovular.

- Binovular twins arise from two fertilized ova, thus each foetus is a separate one with:
  - ➢ Its own amnion and chorion.
  - ➢ Its own sex, though at times the sex may be the same.
  - ➢ Its own genetic make up.

  Thus binovular twins are different in many aspects.
- Uniovular twins are also known as identical or monochorionic or monozygotic. Uniovular twins arise from the same fertilized ovum that has divided itself equally. Thus the foetuses share the same placenta and chorionic membrane but each has its own amniotic membrane. The uniovular twins look alike; they are of the same sex and have the same genetic make up.

# COMPLICATIONS OF MULTIPLE PREGNANCY

The complications of multiple pregnancy can affect the mother and/or her babies during pregnancy, delivery and even after delivery.

- Complications of multiple pregnancy during pregnancy can include:
  - ➢ Increased severity of the minor ailments of pregnancy.
  - ➢ The normal physiological changes during pregnancy are exaggerated.
  - ➢ Pregnancy Induced Hypertension (PIH) is common.

➤ Anaemia common due to increased demand of nutrients like iron and folic acid.
➤ Polyhydramnios.
➤ Antepartum haemorrhage, especially placenta praevia is common due to the bigger placental area compared to singleton pregnancies.
➤ Spontaneous abortion.
➤ Preterm labour.

> **MULTIPLE PREGNANCY DOES NOT USUALLY GO BEYOND THE EXPECTED DATE OF DELIVERY.**

➤ Congenital malformations are more common in multiple pregnancies then singletons. Neural tubal defects, cardiac abnormalities and incidences of. Turner's syndrome and Klinefelter's syndromes are all increased.
➤ Transfusion baby syndrome. This is a condition common in uniovular twinning when there is a communicating blood vessel in the placenta. In this state one foetus can get reduced blood supply and thus it will get fewer nutrients and therefore its growth will be retarded. The other foetus may be getting more blood supply and thus excessive nutrients and therefore becomes bulky, plethoric and polycythemic. At times the baby deprived of nutrients dies early in the uterus and becomes dehydrated and mummified (foetus papyraceous or compressus).
➤ Fusion of the babies (Siamese twins). The fusion can be at any level and of any severity.
• Complications of multiple pregnancy could include:
➤ Labour. If labour gets prolonged a problem should be suspected.

➢ The foetuses may be locked or conjoint. This may be so if the first twin is breech while the second is transverse, or if both babies present as cephalic.

➢ Postpartum haemorrhage (PPH) due to the large placental bed, over-distension of the uterus and uterine inertia.

➢ Retained second twin.

➢ Increased perinatal mortality, especially of the second and subsequent babies.

• The complications of multiple pregnancy after delivery include:

➢ Postpartum haemorrhage (PPH) due to the large placental bed, over-distension of the uterus and uterine inertia.

➢ Poor feeding of the babies. Usually the milk produced by the woman is enough for only one baby; thus there will be a need to give milk supplements for the born babies. It is financially expensive to feed the babies.

➢ Due to feeding problems the babies can get protein-energy malnutrition.

# MANAGEMENT OF MULTIPLE PREGNANCY

Due to the complications of multiple pregnancy, as listed earlier, multiple pregnancy needs careful management during pregnancy, labour and thereafter.

• During pregnancy a woman with multiple pregnancy should be:

➢ Advised to increase food intake. The patient should be given fersolate and folic acid, routinely. This is to make sure the babies get enough nutrients and the mother's haemoglobin rises.

➢ Encouraged to rest more often so as to increase placental blood flow.

➢ Admitted to hospital. It used to be advised that such patients should be admitted to hospital from 32–34 weeks of gestation until delivery. This was believed that it reduces the risk of preterm labour. Many studies have disproved this thus patients are admitted into hospital if other conditions like PPH, pretem labour arise.

➢ Ultrasound of the babies should be repeated around 36 weeks of gestation so as to determine the lie of the babies and decide the mode of delivery.

Delivery should be by caesarean section if:

✓ The first baby is transverse.

✓ The first baby is breech while the second is transverse.

✓ The first baby is breech while the second is cephalic.

✓ Both babies are breech.

✓ More than two babies.

Otherwise vaginal delivery is preferred.

• During labour.

Occasionally a Clinical Officer/midwife may be forced to manage such patients in labour at health centre because either the patient did not take the advice of referral or she comes as an undiagnosed case; thus it is important for a Clinical Officer/midwife to have the skills of managing such patients.

Labour of a woman with multiple pregnancy should be allowed to progress normally. Usually the labour is not prolonged. If labour gets prolonged then there is an undiagnosed problem like locked twins, conjoint twins or first baby is in transverse lie so the patient should be referred to hospital immediately. The delivery of the first baby is usually difficulty. The membrane should not be ruptured until the first baby is delivered. As soon as the first baby is delivered, the following should be done:

> The delivered baby should be handed to an assistant for resuscitation.
> The heart of the second foetus should be auscultated.
> The lie and presentation of the foetus should be determined by abdominal palpation. If the foetal lie is transverse external cephalic version (E.C.V.) should be performed. If E.C.V. is difficult the membranes should immediately be ruptured and internal podalic version and breech extraction performed immediately.
> If the lie is longitudinal the membranes should immediately be ruptured. If breech presents then the author prefers to do breech extraction immediately. If the foetus presents with cephalic the mother should be encouraged to bear down. Sometimes the uterus goes into inertia; thus the uterus should be stimulated with syntocinon. It is for this uterine inertia that the author prefers to set a drip of plain 5% Dextrose at the onset of labour. The drip is allowed to run at a slow rate. Syntocinon 5–10 i.u. is added immediately after the first baby is born and the drip's speed increased to about 40 drops per minute.
> If the second baby is not born fast, high vacuum extraction could be performed.

THE SECOND BABY SHOULD JOIN THE COT OF THE FIRST BABY WITHIN 20 MINUTES.

> Immediately after delivery of the second baby is handed to the assistant. The uterine cavity is explored to rule out another undiagnosed baby.
> If there is no other foetus in the uterus the third stage of labour should be managed actively so as to prevent PPH.

# RETAINED SECOND TWIN

The second twin is said to be retained if it is not delivered within one hour from delivery of the first baby. The causes of retained second twin include:

- Delaying the delivery of the second twin.
- Injecting ergometrine to the mother before delivery of the second twin.

## Management of retained second twin

Management of retained second twin depends on whether the baby is alive or dead.

If the baby is dead augment labour with Syntocinon and allow the baby to be delivered vaginally. If the foetus is alive refer the patient to hospital for further management.

---

RETAINED SECOND TWIN USUALLY INDICATES BAD MIDWIFERY TECHNIQUE.

---

The newborn babies need careful supervision. The babies need iron supplements as they can develop iron deficiencies with ease. Parents of the babies should be advised on family planning so as to have a long period of caring for their babies before the next pregnancy.

# CHAPTER 10

# ANTEPARTUM HAEMORRHAGE (A.P.H)

## INTRODUCTION

Antepartum haemorrhage is a common abnormality in pregnancy. It is a condition, which can be easily mismanaged as it might present in a mild form only to lead into a fatal state. A Clinical Officer/midwife is not supposed to manage this condition but he/she should be able to:
- Define A.P.H and its major types.
- Diagnose and transfer, safely, patients with A.P.H.
- Differentiate between the major types of A.P.H.

## DEFINITION OF A.P.H

Antepartum haemorrhage is bleeding per vaginum from the 24th week of gestation to delivery of the baby.

## CAUSES OF A.P.H

The causes of A.P.H can be grouped into:
- Local causes of APH include:
  ➢ Bleeding from the vulva due to ruptured vulval varicose veins.

> Bleeding from the vagina due to vaginitis.
> Bleeding from the cervix due to:
 ✓ Cervical polyp.
 ✓ Cervical cancer.
 ✓ Cervical erosion.
 ✓ Cervicitis
• Major causes of APH. There are mainly three major causes of APH.
> Placenta praevia.
> Abruption placenta.
> Indeterminate.

The following discussion is on the major causes. Note that a heavy show may be confused with A.P.H., but in show the blood will be mixed with a mucoid discharge.

# PLACENTA PRAEVIA

## Definition

Placenta praevia is defined as bleeding per vaginum due to separation of an abnormally situated placenta, from the $24^{th}$ week of gestation to delivery of the baby. Normally, the placenta is situated in the upper segment of the uterus and commonly at the fundus. A placenta situated in the lower part (lower segment) of the uterus is said to be abnormally situated.

## Types of Placenta praevia

Placenta praevia used to be clinically graded into four types, fig.–14. With the advent of ultrasound the placenta praevia is graded as marginal (grade I), lateral (grade II = touching the cervix but not crossing it) or central (grade III = crossing the cervix when closed and grade IV = covering the cervix even when open).

## Clinical features of Placenta praevia

Suggestive clinical features include:
- Patient complaining of painless vaginal bleeding that is bleeding not accompanied by abdominal pain. This clinical picture is very important even if the patient is not bleeding at the time of seeing her. The bleeding may coincide with onset of labour.
- Abnormal presentation of the foetus, especially breech.
- High presenting part at term.
- In placenta praevia usually the abdomen and the uterus are not tender. If the woman is in labour the uterus will be felt to contract and relax. The foetal heart is usually present unless the bleeding has been so severe as to asphyxiate the foetus.

## Investigations for Placenta praevia

The Clinical Officer is not required to carry out any investigations to prove the presence of Placenta praevia because:

> A VAGINAL OR RECTAL EXAMINATION SHOULD NOT BE DONE AT A HEALTH CENTRE OR WARD IN A PATIENT SUSPECTED TO HAVE PLACENTA PRAEVIA.

Sonography can be done if ultrasound is available.

## Transferring a patient with placenta praevia

A Clinical Officer should transfer all patients he/she suspects to have placenta praevia on the basis of the above clinical features discussed. The patient should be referred to hospital immediately even if she is not bleeding or the bleeding is slight because:

> **A SMALL VAGINAL BLEEDING IN A PATIENT WITH PLACENTA PRAEVIA MIGHT BE A WARNING SIGN FOR A HEAVY BLEEDIND IN THE NEAR FUTURE.**

The patient should be resuscitated before transfer. If she is still bleeding or in hypovolaemic shock:

- Sedate her with either Pethidine 100 mg (i/m) intramuscularly or Morphine 15 mg.
- Raise the blood pressure by giving an infusion of normal saline or Ringer's lactate, intravenously and fast.
- Take blood sample, from the patient, for grouping and cross-matching.
- Get suitable donors to accompany her, otherwise blood transfuse the patient immediately if blood is available in the health centre.
- The patient should be transferred to hospital as soon as possible. The patient should be transferred in a lying position with a drip of normal saline or Ringer's lactate, running. A well-trained and equipped midwife should accompany the patient. Remember to transfer the patient with a good referral letter telling the doctor how much the patient bled and the resuscitations done.

In the hospital the following will be done:

- The same resuscitative measures as listed above will be done depending on the patient's condition.
- Ultrasound will be done or repeated.
- If bleeding has stopped.
  - ➤ A gentle speculum examination could be done to rule out any other local cause of vaginal bleeding
  - ➤ No bimanual vaginal examination in the ward.
  - ➤ The patient should be kept in the ward under a close watch as she can start bleeding any time and anywhere. The idea that such patients can be allowed to go home as long as there is no

bleeding is dangerous. The author keeps his patients in the ward under a close watch until they deliver.

➤ The patient should be delivered by 37 or 38 weeks gestation by:

✓ Elective Lower segment caesarean section (LSCS) in grades II–IV.

✓ In grade I induction with either syntocinon or prostaglandin is recommended.

• If the bleeding does not stop and the maternal condition is threatened the pregnancy should be terminated by performing LCSC.

## Causes of Placenta praevia

• Mostly not known.
• Parity. It is more common in multiparous women than in primigravida.
• Multiple pregnancy (here the common reason is due to the big size of the placenta and or many placentae).
• Uterine fibroid, especially submucus type.

The vaginal bleeding in this abnormally implanted placenta is commonly due to:

➤ The shearing stress between the placenta and the lower segment as the latter stretches.

➤ Trauma especially coitus and vaginal examination can start the bleeding.

## Complications of Placenta praevia

The complications for placenta praevia depend on the severity of the bleeding. The complications could be maternal, foetal or both.

• Maternal complications include:

➤ Hypovolaemic shock, especially when the bleeding is sudden and severe.

- ➢ Anaemia.
- ➢ Postpartum haemorrhage. This is due to the failure of the lower segment to retract after delivery of the placenta.
- ➢ Postpartum infection. This is mainly due to anaemia (an anaemic woman can easily be infected) or vaginal manipulations and/or operative delivery.
- Foetal complications include:
  - ➢ Preterm especially when delivery is forced prematurely due to severity of the bleeding or wrong dates.
  - ➢ Intra-uterine foetal death. This complication occurs if the placenta separates before delivery of the foetus or if there is severe maternal anaemia.
  - ➢ Foetal abnormality. The cause or effect of this is not well known.

# ABRUPTIO PLACENTA

## Definition

Abruptio placenta is bleeding per vaginum due to separation of a normally implanted placenta from the 24th week of gestation to delivery of the baby. The other terms of abruption placenta are accidental haemorrhage and abruptio placenta.

## Types of Abruptio placenta

Abruptio placenta can be:

- Concealed. This is premature separation of the placenta but all blood is hidden behind the placenta as a retro-placental clot and no bleeding is seen per vaginum. In this situation there is no outlet for the retro-placental bleeding.

- Revealed That is, some blood is seen coming out per vaginum. In this state it means there is an outlet for the retro-placental blood.
- Mixed type i.e. some blood is found at the retro-placental space and some is seen coming out per vaginum. This is the commonest type of abruptio placenta encountered in practice.

## Clinical features of Abruptio placenta

Suggestive clinical features of abruptio placenta include:
- Patient complaining of sudden onset of abdominal pains.
- Patient complaining of vaginal bleeding if abruptio placenta is the mixed or revealed type. In the absence of vaginal bleeding, as in concealed abruption placenta, other causes of sudden abdominal pains should be thought of. In the presence of vaginal bleeding still other causes of abdominal pains like ruptured uterus, should be thought of.
- The blood is non-clotting.
- The patient might look more pale and shocked than can be explained by the amount of blood lost per vaginum. This is due to some of the concealed blood in the retro-placental area.
- The abdomen and uterus are usually tender and hard due to uterine spasms.
- The uterus does not relax as it is in constant spasms.
- Many times the foetal heart is not heard as the foetus is dead.
- Foetal parts are hard to feel due to tenderness of the abdomen and the uterine spasms.

## Investigation

For a Clinical Officer there is no specific investigation he/she can do. The final diagnosis is at delivery when a retro-placental clot is seen. In centres where sonography can be done, this can help clinch the diagnosis.

## Management

The patient should be referred to hospital as soon as possible. If blood is available the patient should be transfused otherwise a plasma expander should be set up or if not available normal saline drip should be set up. A continuous bladder catheter should be inserted. In the hospital:

- The patient should be resuscitated quickly, as in placenta praevia. Blood should be looked for and the patient should be transfused immediately. If blood is not available immediately frozen plasma should be given.
- Delivery should be effect as soon as possible by setting up Syntocinon drip.
- Amniotomy should be performed.

> **REMOVE THE OFFENDING PLACENTA AS SOON AS POSSIBLE.**

The prognosis of the patient depends on the time taken to deliver her. Vaginal delivery is safer than caesarean section due to the high bleeding tendency of such patients. If the baby is alive and blood is available a gynaecologist can perform a fast caesarean section. The operation should not be done by a junior doctor as the maternal and perinatal mortality rates could be very high. The author is hesitant to perform caesarean section as many times the patients have massive abruption placenta and such an operation does not reduce the perinatal mortality but increases the maternal morbidity and mortality.

## Causes of Abruption placentae

As in placenta praevia, the causes of abruption placenta are mostly not known. Factors, which can predispose a woman to get abruption placenta, include:

- Severe physical or mental stress.

- Hypertensive diseases in pregnancy (including PIH/eclampsia).
- High parity.
- Advanced maternal age.
- When the liquor is allowed to drain suddenly.

## Complications of Abruption placenta

The complications of abruptio placenta are either foetal, maternal or both.
- Maternal complications include:
  - ➤ Anaemia.
  - ➤ If amniotic fluid or trophoblastic tissue gets into the maternal circulation after a placental abruption this can cause disseminated intra-vascular coagulopathy (DIC), due to depletion of clotting factors. This can lead to bleeding tendency.
  - ➤ Uterine apoplexy. This is when blood of the abruption tracks into the myometrial tissues giving rise to couvelaire uterus. The blood can infiltrate as far as to the peritoneal surface. This can make the uterus not contract effectively.
  - ➤ Postpartum haemorrhage due to depletion of clotting factors, anaemia or couvelaire uterus.
  - ➤ Hypovolaemic shock.
  - ➤ Renal failure due to tubular and glomerular necrosis.
  - ➤ Postpartum infection due to anaemia. Uterine apoplexy, which is infiltration of myometrial muscles with blood giving rise to Couvelaire uterus which cannot contract effectively.
  - ➤ Maternal death.
- Foetal complication is the high perinatal mortality. Many times even if the baby is born alive it dies within the early neonatal life. Many times the abruption is major. Performing an emergency caesarean section for the reason that the foetal heart is heard could just change stillbirth to a neonatal death and at the same time risk the woman to uncontrollable bleeding due to the DIC

# INDETERMINATE A.P.H

Many times the type of A.P.H. is neither of those mentioned earlier thus this is considered as indeterminate A.P.H. This is a post delivery diagnosis.

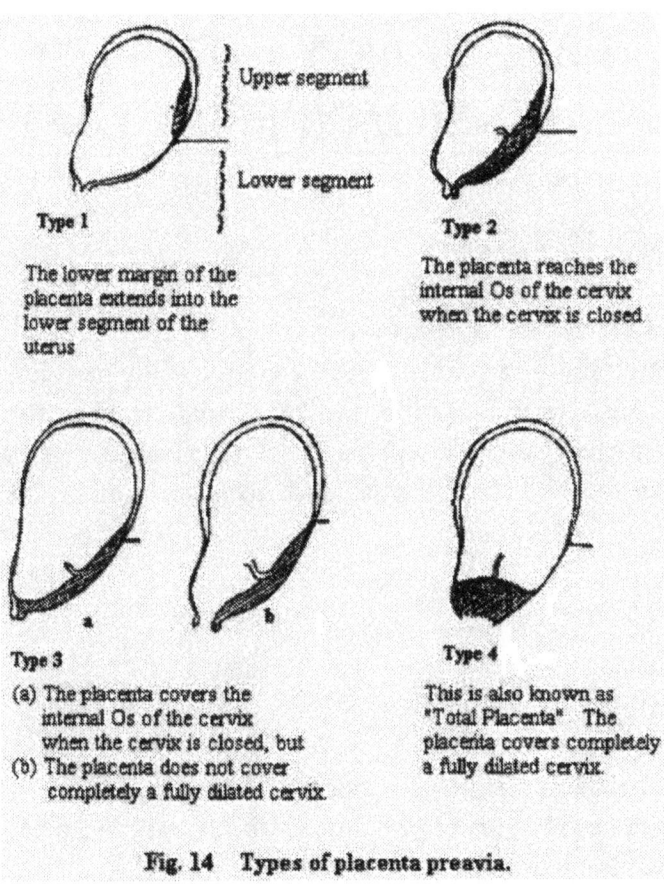

Fig. 14 Types of placenta preavia.

# CHAPTER 11

# PREGNANCY INDUCED HYPERTENSION (PIH)/ECLAMPSIA

## INTRODUCTION

PIH is the second most common problem encountered during pregnancy, labour and puerperium, while anaemia is the first. It is one of the top three causes of maternal mortality worldwide. The other causes of maternal mortality include sepsis and haemorrhage. In Tanzania, PIH is common along the coastal areas and not common in the cold hilly areas!

## OBJECTIVES

The student is expected to be able to:
- Define PIH.
- List the classification of hypertension in pregnancy.
- Diagnose PIH during pregnancy, labour and puerperium.
- Detect the women at risk of developing PIH.
- Manage patients with PIH.
- List the complications of PIH.
- Discuss HELLP syndrome.
- Define eclampsia.
- Diagnose eclampsia.

- Give first aid care to an eclamptic patient.
- Prevent eclampsia.

# DEFINITION OF PIH

PIH is a condition characterized by oedema, proteinuria and hypertension during pregnancy from the 20th week. PIH is also known as "the specific hypertensive disease of pregnancy", EPH (oedema, protein hypertension) gestosis and pre-eclampsia (PE). The old term of PIH was pre-eclampsia toxaemia (P.E.T).

# CASSIFICATION OF HYPERTENSION IN PREGNANCY

## Pregnancy induced hypertension

See definition above. Any two of the three main characteristics of PIH after the gestation period of 20 weeks are enough to diagnose PIH.

- Oedema of the legs, sacral area, and anterior abdomen or of fingers is one of the main clinical features of PIH. Oedema (especially of the ankles) is often seen during pregnancy in about 30% of pregnant women without being an abnormal occurrence. Oedema existing on its own can be called "good" as it may mean that a big foetus is present.
- Proteinuria. This is presence of protein in urine. Proteinuria is a bad sign as it shows that the disease has spread. The presence of proteinuria, which is not due to U.T.1, is a very bad sign as the foetal prognosis is worsened by 10%. The presence of protein greater than 0.5 gm in 24 hours urine or greater than 300mg/ml of urine (+ dipstick) is bad. The longer and the higher the proteinuria the worse the foetal prognosis.

• Hypertension is also a bad sign. A blood pressure of 140/90mm Hg or more during any time of pregnancy indicates hypertension. A rise of systolic blood pressure of 30 mm Hg or diastolic blood pressure of 15 mm Hg or more above the pre-pregnant level indicates hypertension. The raised blood pressure should persist after 4–6 hours of bed rest.

Apart from the aforesaid major clinical features indicating PIH, excessive weight gains of 1.0 kg or more in any one week of pregnancy is significant for PIH.

Patients with PIH usually have no complaints unless the condition is severe. In severe PIH the patient might complain of frontal headache, epigastric pain, seeing stars in the eyes and/or vomiting.

## Chronic hypertension

This is diagnosed if blood press is 140/90 mm. Hg. or more before pregnancy, before 20 weeks of pregnancy or if it persists beyond 42 days after delivery. Chronic hypertension can be essential, idiopathic primary or secondary. These include:
• Essential hypertension (EHT).
• Renal hypertension like:
  ➢ Diabetic glomerulosclerosis.
  ➢ Acute and chronic glomerulonephritis.
  ➢ Polycystic kidney disease.
  ➢ Renal transplant.
• Adrenal hypertension like:
  ➢ Pheocromocytoma.
  ➢ Cushing's diseases and syndrome.
  ➢ Hyperaldosteronism.

- Others may include:
  - ➤ Thyrotoxicosis.
  - ➤ Coarctation of the aorta.

## Chronic hypertension superimposed with PIH

This is diagnosed if in a patient with chronic hypertension the blood pressure increases by at least 30 mm. Hg diastolic or 15 mm Hg. systolic or 20 mm Hg arterial pressure or new onset of proteinuria.

# CAUSES OF PIH

The causes of PIH may be multifactor which include:
- Abnormal trophoblastic invasion of the maternal circulation.
- Altered vascular sensitivity to angiotensin-II.
- Insufficient production of blocking antibodies.
- Endothelial dysfunction.
- Prostaglandin/thromboxane imbalance.
- Genetic predisposition.

# RISK FACTORS FOR DEVELOPMENT OF PIH

- Primiparity.
  Generally, PIH is a disease of first pregnancy (primigravida). A previous normal pregnancy, even if it was an abortion, is associated with a markedly lowered incidence of PIH.

- Paternity.
  - ➤ The protective effect of multiparity is lost with change of partner.
  - ➤ A partner who fathered a PIH pregnancy in another woman increases the chance of his new partner developing PIH.

- Previous PIH, age and interval between pregnancies.
  A patient with PIH stands a high chance of developing PIH in subsequent pregnancies. Increase maternal age and long intervals between pregnancies increases the risk of developing PIH.
- Family history of PIH increases the chances of developing PIH.
- Underlying disorders like:
  ➤ Chronic hypertension.
  ➤ Renal diseases.
  ➤ Obesity.
  ➤ Diabetes mellitus.
  ➤ Thrombophilic disorders.
- Pregnancy associated risks like multiple pregnancy and hydatid-form mole.
- Psychosocial strain, physical and mental strain.

# EFFECTS OF PIH

PIH is a multisystemic disease. It can involve:
- The brain.
  ➤ Cerebral oedema.
  ➤ Cerebral haemorrhage.
  ➤ Cerebral infarction.
  The patient can be unconscious or coma.
- Eyes.
  ➤ Papilloedema.
  ➤ Retinal detachment.
  ➤ Cortical blindness.
- Liver.
  ➤ Congestion.
  ➤ Haemorrhage.
  ➤ Infarction

➢ Rupture.

The patient may complain of epigastric pain, liver function tests may be abnormal. In haemorrhage the patient may be anaemic.

- Blood.
  - ➢ Thrombocytopenia.
  - ➢ DIC.
- Lungs.
  - ➢ Pulmonary oedema.
  - ➢ Aspiration pneumonia especially during convulsions.
- Reproductive.
  - ➢ Intra-uterine foetal growth retardation (IUFGR).
  - ➢ Foetal death.
  - ➢ Preterm delivery.
  - ➢ Abruptio placenta.
- Mucosa leading to laryngeal oedema.
- Skin.
  - ➢ Oedema.
  - ➢ Petechial haemorrhage.
  - ➢ Ecchymosis.

# COMPLICATIONS OF PIH

Any of the systems listed above if involved severely will cause complication to the mother, baby or both.

- Common foetal complications include prematurity intra-uterine foetal growth retardation (IUGR), foetal distress, intra-uterine foetal death (IUD), stillbirths and neonatal death. The perinatal morbidity and mortality are high.
- Common maternal complications include eclampsia (discussed later), cerebral vascular accident, and abruption placenta; subcapsular haemorrhage of the liver heart and renal failure.

- HELLP syndrome. Help develops in patients with severe PIH or eclampsia.
  The acronym of HELLP is:
  - ➢ H = Haemolysis. There will be decreased haematocrit, low haemoglobin, increased reticulocytes and increased bilirubin.
  - ➢ EL = Elevated Liver Enzymes. Enzymes like, alkaline phosphatase, SGOT and SGPT.
  - ➢ LP = Low platelet count (thrombocytopenia). This is used to classify HELLP syndrome as:
    - ✓ Class I. Platelets are 50,000 cells/µl or less. This is severe thrombocytopenia.
    - ✓ Class II. Platelets more than 50,000 cells/µl but not greater than 100,000 cells/µl. This is moderate thrombocytopenia.
    - ✓ Class III. Platelets more than 100,000 cells/µl but less than 150,000 cells/µl. This is mild thrombocytopenia.

Conditions like viral hepatitis, acute fatty liver, cholecystitis and many others should be ruled out.

## GRADES OF PIH

PIH used to be graded into mild moderate and severe. It is now graded into mild and severe.

- Severe PIH.
  - ➢ Blood pressure of systolic = 160 mm. Hg, or diastolic = 110 mm. Hg, or the both systolic and diastolic pressures =.160/110 mm. Hg. This raised blood pressure should persistent even after 4 6 hours of bed rest.
  - ➢ Proteinuria. = 5 gm of protein in 24 hour urine or dipstick +++ for protein.
  - ➢ Others include:
    - ✓ HELLP syndrome.

✓ Central nervous system dysfunction like blurred vision, scotoma, severe headache.
✓ Epigastric pain or pain in the right upper quadrant of the abdomen.
✓ Oliguria or renal failure.
✓ Eclampsia.
- Mild PIH.

If blood pressure is < 160/110 without any of the other signs of severe PIH then this is graded as mild PIH.

# MANAGEMENT OF PATIENT WITH PIH

The principals of management of PIH are:
- Control blood pressure.
- Prevent eclampsia.
- Delivery.

Management of a patient with PIH depends on the severity of the condition.

## Mild PIH

- During pregnancy.
  ➤ Bed rest.
    Bed rest is usually central to primary management of PIH. This might be the only treatment needed. Bed rest can lower the blood pressure; improve the oedema and nutrient supply to the foetus.

    If there is no accompanying proteinuria or the diastolic blood pressure is < 100 mm. Hg, the systolic blood pressure is < 150 mm. Hg and the patient leaves close to hospital ambulatory management can be tried. The bed rest should take priority over everything else including domestic chores.

If the above conditions are not met it is safer to manage the patient in hospital where bed rest can be reinforced and patient better monitored.

➢ Antihypertensives.
Often then not, antihypertensives will not be needed. If the blood increases despite of good bed rest then antihypertensives should be given. The antihypertensives are mainly to protect the mother from the risk of stroke. The antihypertensives have no effect on the progress of the PIH or on the foetal growth but they help to maintain the pregnancy longer to allow the foetus to become more mature. The antihypertensives include.
   ✓ Methyldopa (Aldomet). This is the commonest antihypertensive used in PIH. The dose is 250–750 mg tid depending on the blood pressure level. Note that aldomet is a slow acting antihypertensive and its peak effect takes 6 8 hours.
   ✓ Other drugs include atenolol (50–100 mg daily), propanolol (20–80 mg tid), labetalol (100–200 mg bid) and nifedipine (10.mg 4–6 hourly).

➢ Diuretics. These are usually of no much use.

DIURETICS ARE NOT NECESSARY IN PIH.

➢ Monitoring. The states of both the mother and foetus should be closely monitored and evaluated.
   ✓ Blood pressure, urine protein and foetal kicks daily.
   ✓ Non-stress test, CBC, blood urea, serum creatinine, uric acid and liver function test weekly. If the non-stress test is

non-reactive biophysical profile of the foetus should be done.

✓ Ultrasound evaluation of foetal growth every 3–4 weeks to determine growth of the foetus and biophysical profile.

• Delivery.
Despite the improvement of PIH the foetus is still at risk. All patients should be delivered by 37 completed weeks of pregnancy.

> PATIENTS WITH PIH SHOULD NOT BE ALLOWED TO GO BEYOND THE EXPECTED DATE OF DELIVERY.

Unless contra indicated vaginal delivery should be attempted in a hospital equipped to perform caesarean section. The patient should therefore be induced (see chapter on induction of labour). During labour the following should be done.

➤ The progress of labour should be monitored very closely. If a partogram is available it should be used.

➤ The state of the foetus should be monitored closely.

✓ Signs of foetal distress should be looked for.

✓ Continuous cardiotocogram if available should be applied otherwise the foetal heart should be monitored every after fifteen minutes.

➤ The state of the mother should be monitored closely.

✓ Blood pressure should be monitored hourly, if possible continuously. The blood pressure might rise or even get worse during labour. If diastolic pressure is 110 mm. Hg or more and or the systolic pressure 160 mm. Hg or more the patient should be given fast acting antihypertensives and magnesium sulphate (see under management of severe PIH).

✓ Urine should be checked for quantity and protein hourly.

- ✓ Signs of impending eclampsia should be looked for and patient should be treated accordingly.
- ➢ Drugs.
  - ✓ 5% Dextrose drip should be set up as the patient has to be kept on nothing per oral until she has delivered.
  - ✓ Sedation with pethidine or diazepam (valium) can be given with caution as they cross the placenta to the foetus. They should not be given if delivery is anticipated to occur within four hours.
  - ✓ The use of Magnesium sulphate for seizure prophylaxis in mild PIH with its risks may out way the benefits.
- • After delivery.
  - ✓ Ergometrine should not be given as it can cause or worsen the blood pressure. If the patient develops postpartum haemorrhage syntocinon is the drug to use.
  - ✓ Maternal condition should be monitored in the ward for at least 48 hours. The first 24 hours are crucial as eclampsia can occur during this period.
  - ✓ Antihypertensives should be continued or started if blood pressure stays high or increases. If the blood pressure continues to be high after 48–72 hours despite of aggressive treatment the patient should be referred to the internist as she might be developing chronic hypertension.
  - ✓ Counselling. The patient should be counselled about future pregnancy. She should be informed the high chances of eat of PIH in subsequent pregnancies and the risk of developing chronic hypertension. Therefore family planning should be discussed and contraception should be advised.
  - ✓ The patient should be seen at postnatal clinic after 4–6 weeks to wean her off the antihypertensives or transfer her to the Hypertension clinic. Also contraception can be provided.

# Severe PIH

Patients discovered to have severe PIH should be referred to hospital immediately. At health centre the clinical officer/midwife can give such a patient pethedine (100.mg i.m stat) or diazepam (10.mg i.m stat) so as to prevent convulsions. Magnesium sulphate, nifedipine or hydralazine (apresoline) should not be given at a health centre. The patient should have an intravenous drip of 5%dextrose.

In the hospital the patient's state will be re assessed.
- Symptoms and signs of impending eclampsia will be looked for.
    - ➤ Persistent occipital or frontal headaches. This may indicate cerebral oedema or haemorrhage.
    - ➤ Right upper quadrant or epigastric pain. This may be due to stretching of liver capsule due to subcapsular congestion, haemorrhage or haematoma.
    - ➤ Visual disturbance like scotoma due to pappiloedema or retinal detachment.
- Investigations to rule out renal damage, HELLP syndrome bleeding and clotting disorders should be done immediately and repeated as necessary.
    - ➤ BUN, creatinine, blood urea, uric acid, urine protein (24 hour urine sample and or dipstick).
    - ➤ Hourly urine output.
    - ➤ CBC, LFT.
    - ➤ Prothrombin test (PT) and Partial Thromboplastin Time (PTT). If facilities are available fibrinogen and fibrinogen degradation products can be estimated.
- The patient should be clinically examined.
    - ➤ Oedema (peripheral and in the lungs).
    - ➤ Abdominally. Epigastric tenderness, fundal height and any other organomegally.

➢ Central nervous system especially, knee reflexes and clonus.
➢ Fundoscopy to rule out pappiloedema.
• The foetus should be assessed.
➢ Non stress test should be done.
➢ Biophysical profile (amniotic fluid index, foetal muscle tone, foetal body movements, foetal breathing and heart beat).

The management of a patient with severe hypertension should be in a hospital with both obstetrical and neonatal facilities preferable with intensive care facilities. Traditionally women with severe PIH had been delivered immediately regardless of the foetal consideration. In centres where the maternal condition can be monitored closely, a patient with severe PIH can be managed in one of the two ways.

• Expectant management.
  It is true that each week gained in utero confers tangible benefit to the neonatal outcome. In the past when infants born before 30 weeks rarely survived it made no sense to manage severe PIH expectantly before 28 weeks of gestation. Due to the improvement of monitoring maternal and foetal well-being and improvement of neonatal resuscitation technology severe PIH presenting at 24–26 weeks of gestation can be managed conservatively! Selection of such patients will depend on both maternal and foetal condition. Certainly maternal condition takes precedence over the foetal condition.
  ➢ Foetal conditions for expectant management.
    ✓ Reactive non stress test with no repetitive late or severe decelerations.
    ✓ Biophysical profile greater than 4.
    ✓ Amniotic fluid index greater than 7 cm.
    ✓ Ultrasound estimated weight above the 5th percentile.
    ✓ Gestation period less than 32 weeks.
  ➢ Maternal conditions for expectant management.

    ✓ Controlled hypertension.
    ✓ Normal urine output.
    ✓ No tenderness over the right upper quadrant of the abdomen.

The expectant management will include.
➤ Treatment.
    ✓ Bed rest. The patient should be nursed in a quiet place with no flickering lights. The patient should be close to the nursing station so as to monitor her with ease.
    ✓ Control blood pressure.
    If diastolic blood pressure is 110 mm. Hg or more its should be lowered by either nifedipine (10 mg sublingually then 10 mg 6 hourly for 24–48 hours depending on the blood pressure response. It should not be administered if the diastolic blood pressure is less than 100 mm. Hg) or apresoline (5 mg i.v stat or 50 mg in 500 mls 5%dextrose titrated in accordance to the blood pressure response. Also apresoline should not be given if the diastolic blood pressure is less than 100 mm. Hg). The author adds aldomet 1000 mg stat the 500–750 mg (depending on diastolic blood pressure) tid with the expectation that the patient's blood pressure will be controlled within 48 hours and thus be maintained on methyldopa when the diastolic blood pressure is less 100 mm. Hg. The nifedipine/apresoline is given whenever necessary.
    ✓ Prevent convulsions/eclampsia.
    The first line anticonvulsant is Magnesium sulphate (see administration of magnesium sulphate in the treatment/prevention of eclampsia. Other drugs include diazepam and pethidine.

✓ Lung maturity. If the foetal maturity is less then 32 weeks it is advisable to give the mother corticosteroid therapy (two doses of dexamethazone 12 mg i.m. 12 hourly) so as to mature the foetal lungs

➢ Monitoring maternal and foetal states as stated under mild PIH, but more frequently.

• Expeditious delivery.
Delivery should be done within 72 hours in the following states.
➢ Foetal conditions.
    ✓ Gestation period is 34 or more weeks.
    ✓ Biophysical profile more than 4.
    ✓ Severe IUGR.
    ✓ Repetitive late or severe variable deceleration.
    ✓ Severe oligohydramnios.
➢ Maternal conditions.
    ✓ Uncontrolled severe hypertension within 48–72 hours.
    ✓ HELLP syndrome especially when the red blood cells less than 100,000/ µl.
    ✓ Raised liver enzymes with epigastric pain or right upper quadrant tenderness.
    ✓ Symptoms and signs of impending eclampsia.
    ✓ Oliguria.
    ✓ Pulmonary oedema.
    ✓ Persistent headache or visual changes.
    ✓ Abruption placenta.
    ✓ Eclampsia.

Delivery is as said under mild PIH. Drugs to lower the blood pressure and prevent eclampsia as said above should be instituted. Vaginal delivery is preferred to elective caesarean section unless contraindicated. Post delivery management and advice on family planning is as in mild PIH.

## Treatment of HELLP syndrome

These patients usually have severe PIH but have special needs above the treatment of the severe PIH.

- Blood pressure should be controlled if severe.
- Magnesium sulphate should be given both during and after delivery so as to control eclampsia
- Body fluids and electrolytes should be maintained by giving the appropriate intravenous fluids like 5% Dextrose alternating with Normal saline and Ringer's lactate.
- If the platelet count is less than 50,000 per μl or the patient is bleeding the patient should be transfused with fresh blood, preferably platelets.
- Patients with platelets less than 100,000 per μl should be given high doses of corticosteroids like dexamethasone. This may eliminate the need to blood transfuse the patient.

# ECLAMPSIA

Eclampsia is characterized by fits (convulsions) like those of grand-mal epilepsy and/or coma superimposed upon PIH. Eclampsia can occur during pregnancy, labour or within the first 24 hours of puerperium. During eclampsia there is an intense vasospasm with tissue anoxia. Cerebral anoxia can cause convulsions and/or coma. During eclampsia the uterine blood flow is further reduced, as is the renal blood flow and consequently glomerular filtration rate is decreased and urinary output decreased. About 50% of eclampsia occurs during pregnancy, 30% during labour and 20% after delivery.

## Clinical features of eclampsia

Eclampsia is usually preceded by a period of deterioration of PIH called "imminent eclampsia". In about 20% of patients eclampsia occurs with very little warning. If the period of imminent eclampsia is not recognized, and treated immediately, fits will develop. The fits have three stages:

- Premonitory or aura stage. In this stage the patient rolls her eyes and starts twitching her hands and/or face.
- Tonic stage. This stage is characterized by spreading muscular spasms until the patient is rigid. During the tonic stage cyanosis is intense due to fixation of the chest and diaphragm.
- Clonus stage. This stage is characterized by rapid and spasmodic muscular contractions. The patient breathes torturously and bubbly. The patient later goes into a coma. The fits may however continue and unless controlled may end in the death of the foetus and/or mother.
- The reflexes like knee reflex are usually exaggerated.

## Differential diagnosis of eclampsia

Eclampsia is the most common cause of coma during pregnancy.

UNTILL PROVED OTHERWISE A COMATOUS PREGNANT PATIENT HAS ECLAMPSIA.

Other diseases that can cause coma during pregnancy include:

- Epilepsy. Epilepsy is not associated with hypertension, proteinuria or hyper-reflexia.
- Cerebral haemorrhage due to other cause or any space occupying lesion. In these conditions hypertension may be present. If in doubt lumbar puncture can be done under sedation and if the cerebral spinal fluid contains blood, cerebral haemorrhage may be

suspected. In eclampsia the cerebrospinal fluid is usually clear and normal.

- Diabetic coma. In this condition blood sugar is high.
- Uraemia. Uraemia may be due to renal failure, which is one of the complications of eclampsia. The blood urea and uric acid are high.

## Complications of eclampsia

Eclampsia is a dreadful condition associated with high maternal and perinatal mortality and morbidity.

- Maternal complications of eclampsia include pulmonary oedema, hyper-pyrexia, renal failure, cardiac failure and cerebral vascular accident. A woman who has had eclampsia has a high chance of developing hypertension later in life.
- Foetal complications include stillbirths, neonatal death, foetal distress and prematurity.

## Treatment of eclampsia

Eclampsia is an emergency condition. The more fits the patient gets the higher the maternal and perinatal mortality or morbidity. The number of fits depends on the efficiency of treatment. All eclamptics should be referred to hospital. Before referring the patient the Clinical Officer should resuscitate the patient by:

- Clear airway. Insert a mouth gag (a well-padded metal spatula is useful) to prevent her from biting her tongue during a fit. Suck secretions from her mouth and trachea/oesophagus. Give her oxygen.
- Control and prevent convulsions by giving anyone of the anticonvulsants in high doses like diazepam 20 mg intravenously as a bolus and then set up a drip of 5% dextrose 500 mls add 20–40 mg of diazepam and run it at 30–40 drops/min; Phenytoin 200

mg i.m 4–6 hourly or Lytic cocktail of Pethidine 100 mg and Promethazine 50 mg given intravenously or intramuscularly. Magnesium sulphate is the drug of choice recommended by W.H.O. Such a drug should not be used at health centre level for fear of its side effects. Many eclamptic convulsions will resolve spontaneously in 60–90 seconds. It is unwise and potentially dangerous to abolish or shorten the seizure activity. After the convulsion has ended then an initial dose of the anticonvulsant can be given.

- A drip of 5% Dextrose should be set up with a wide bored cannula.

When the convulsions have been controlled, the patient can then be transferred to hospital. A nurse equipped to control further convulsions and/or assist delivery should escort the patient.

## Management of eclampsia in hospital

The aims of treatment of an eclamptic patient are to clear airway, stop/prevent fits, deliver, management of unconsciousness and preventing complications.

- Resuscitation.
  - ➤ Clear airway as said above.
  - ➤ Control and prevent further convulsions as said above. Magnesium sulphate can be used (see under administration of Magnesium sulphate in the treatment/prevention of eclampsia).
  - ➤ The patient should be nursed in a semi-prone position. The patient's bed should be close to the nurse's office and the room should be well lit. The lights should not be flickering or switched on and off as this might trigger a convulsion. The room should be quiet.

> These patients are better managed in an intensive care unit.
> If the blood pressure is dangerously high it should be lowered by giving apresoline as said under severe PIH.
> Investigations as said under management of severe PIH should be done immediately but they should not delay the final management which is delivery.

- Delivery.
  After the convulsions have been controlled and the blood pressure lowered the foetus should be delivered as soon as possible regardless of its maturity. The condition usually settles after delivery of the placenta! Note that each convulsion increases maternal mortality and morbidity accumulatively. Therefore delivery should not be delayed. Unless vaginal delivery is imminent the patient should undergo caesarean section as soon as possible.

- Post delivery management.
  > Intravenous fluids should be continued for at least 24 hours. Continuous urine drainage for at least 24 hours. Hourly urine output should be recorded. Therefore fluid input and output should be monitored closely. Blood pressure and pulse should be monitored hourly. Signs of renal failure, liver failure and cerebral vascular accident should be looked for.
  > All the other tests done pre-delivery should be repeated post delivery.
  > Anticonvulsants should be continued for at least 24 hours.
  > The patient should remain in hospital for at least 48 hours.
  > The patients should be advised about family planning and be seen in postnatal clinic.

# ADMINISTRATION OF MAGNESSIUM SULPHATE

Magnesium sulphate is the first line drug for the treatment and prevention of eclampsia recommended by W.H.O.

## Dosage

The dose does not vary with patient's weight or body mass. There are different regimes used like Pritchard's, Zuspan's and Sibai's. Each centre has to decide which regime or combination to use. In St. Jude hospital, St. Lucia the following regime is in use.

- Initial dose/loading dose.
    - ➢ Intravenously. 4–5 gms. Magnesium sulphate is diluted in 100 mls 5% Dextrose and given intravenously slowly for 15–20 minutes.

        Or

    - ➢ Intramuscularly. 10 gms of Magnesium sulphate is diluted in 10 mls of 5% Dextrose. Half of it is injected into each buttock with 1.0 ml of 2% xylocaine or lignocaine.

    If convulsions persist after 15 minutes an additional of 2.0 gms of Magnesium sulphate can be given as a bolus over five minutes. Most women will remain seizure free for a long time after the loading dose.

- Maintenance dose.

    A continuous infusion of Magnesium sulphate is given via an infusion at the rate of 1.0 gm per hour or 4 gms of the Magnesium sulphate is injected intramuscularly as in the loading dose but four hourly. If the patient's condition improves or she delivers then the maintenance dose can be stopped after 24 hours

# Prerequisites for administration of Magnesium sulphate

- Urine output should not be less than 30 mls. per hour.
- Respiratory rate should not be less than 12 per hour.
- Deep tendon reflexes, especially tendon reflex should be positive.
- Maternal blood pressure and pulse should be monitored.
- 10% Calcium gluconate should be available for treatment of Magnesium sulphate toxicity.

# Side effects of Magnesium sulphate

The therapeutic and toxic doses are very close.
- Loss of patellar reflex.
- Muscular paralysis.
- Respiratory arrest.
- Cardiac arrest.
- Decreased uterine contractions thus PPH can occur.
- Depression of neonatal neuromuscular and respiratory activities.
- Anaesthetic complications.

# CHAPTER 12

# POLYHYDRAMNIOS

## INTRODUCTION

Polyhydramnios is not a very common condition. Polyhydramnios has a clinical importance because of the conditions associated with it, the distress it may produce, the difficulties it causes in abdominal examination and the ill effects it may exert on the course of labour and after.

## OBJECTIVES

The student should be able to:
- Define polyhydramnios.
- Diagnose polyhydramnios.
- List the possible causes of polyhydramnios.
- List the complications of polyhydramnios.
- Refer to hospital a patient with polyhydramnios.

## DEFINITION

Polyhydramnios is also known as hydramnios. Polyhydramnios means excessive liquor; more than 1500mls. The normal amount of liquor is 300–800 mls. When the liquor is less than 300mls this is called oligohydramnios. Sonographically an amniotic fluid index greater than 20 is considered as polyhydramnios while if the index is less 7 is oligohydramnios.

# CIRCULATION OF LIQUOR

In early pregnancy the composition of liquor closely resembles that of maternal plasma.

## Production of liquor

- Foetal skin in early pregnancy, to 18 weeks, is permeable to water; so that the liquor has been regarded as the largest part of foetal extra-cellular fluid. After 18 weeks of pregnancy the foetal skin is impermeable to water.
- The umbilical cord may also produce its exudates.
- Between 12–14 weeks of pregnancy the foetal kidneys begin to function and the foetus begins to urinate. Urine contributes considerably to the liquor.
- Tracheal fluids also contribute to the liquor.
- The amniotic membranes also contribute to the liquor.

## Absorption of liquor

- The foetus, at term, swallows a lot of the liquor, about 210–760 mls per day.
- The foetal skin in early pregnancy is also permeable to water.
- The foetal surface of the placenta can absorb liquor.
- The lungs of the foetus absorb liquor.
- The umbilical cord may absorb some liquor.

# CAUSES OF POLYHYDRAMNIOS

The cause of polyhydramnios is an excess formation over absorption of liquor.

In 50% of the patients, polyhydramnios may owe its origin to maternal or foetal causes or both.

- Maternal causes include:
  - ➤ It is commoner in multiparous than in primigravidae.
  - ➤ Diabetes mellitus.
  - ➤ Congestive cardiac failure.
  - ➤ PIH.
- Foetal causes include:
  - ➤ Multiple pregnancy, especially of the uniovular type.
  - ➤ Foetal abnormality like anencephaly, oesophageal atresia, spina bifida and hydrocephalus.
  - ➤ Other foetal conditions include hydrops foetalis and chorioangioma.

# CLINICAL FEATURES OF POLYHYDRAMNIOS

## Symptoms

In gradual onset type of polyhydramnios the patient may complain of:
- Unmanageable abdominal girth.
- Shortness of breath.
- Increasingly troublesome varicose veins.
- Oedema of ankles.
- Tense abdomen.

## Signs

The patient may be:

- Restless.
- Dyspnoeic.
- Pitting oedema of both legs.
- The abdominal skin may look shiny.
- Fluid thrill is positive while shifting dullness is negative.
- The foetal heartbeat may be distant.
- The foetal parts may be hard to palpate.
- Malpresentation and abnormal lies of the foetus.

## Investigations

In a health centre there are few, if any, investigations to prove the presence of polyhydramnios. The Clinical Officer has to depend on clinical features. If there are radiological facilities then an abdominal X-ray can be taken and the baby will look smaller than the size of the uterus. The X-ray will may also show the presence of twins and skeletal foetal abnormalities as listed earlier. In centres with ultrasound machines sonography is preferred to X-raying.

# DIFFERENTIAL DIAGNOSIS OF POLYHYDRAMNIOS

Polyhydramnios should be differentiated from other causes where the uterus is bigger than dates in:
- Wrong dates or more advanced pregnancy than indicated by menstrual history.
- Multiple pregnancy without polyhydramnios.
- Fibroids or ovarian cysts complicating pregnancy.
- An unusually large foetus.
- Gaseous distension of bowel in association with partial or intermittent colonic obstruction in the chronic air sallower.

- Hydatidform mole.
- Full bladder.

# COMPLICATIONS OF POLYHYDRAMNIOS

Polyhydramnios is associated with complication during:
- Pregnancy where there could be preterm delivery especially in. acute states. There could be foetal abnormal lie or malpresentation due to the greater foetal mobility in the uterus. Premature rupture of membranes; accompanied by intra-uterine infection or prolapse of the cord or arm.
- During labour there is an increased risk of abruptio placenta if the liquor escapes too rapidly. There is high incidence of postpartum haemorrhage due to associated uterine inertia.

# MANAGEMENT OF POLYHYDRAMNIOS

All patients diagnosed to have polyhydramnios should be referred to hospital, immediately, for investigation and treatment. Such patients need to be relieved of their discomforts by:
- Bed rest. They should lie propped up and not supine, to avoid supine hypotensive syndrome.
- They may need analgesics and if necessary sedatives to ensure sleep.
- Diuretics can occasionally be given to keep the condition in check though this treatment will not reduce the volume of fluid present.
- In more severe degrees of polyhydramnios amniocentesis can be tried. The author prefers to observe the patients in hospital until they go into spontaneous labour as many times they go into preterm labour.
- Indomethacin has been found to reduce the amniotic liquor.

A PREGNANCY COMPLICATED WITH POLYHYDRAMNIOS DOES NOT GO BEYOND THE EXPECTED DATE OF DELIVERY.

The third stage of labour should be managed actively and the baby should be examined, thoroughly to rule out any congenital malformations, before the first feed.

# CHAPTER 13

# MEDICAL DISEASES IN PREGNANCY

## INTRODUCTION

A pregnant woman is not immune to getting any medical disease. There are certain medical conditions, which are common during pregnancy. These conditions either appear commonly in pregnancy or pregnancy worsens them. The common medical diseases are anaemia, urinary tract infection, malaria, diabetes mellitus and cardiac diseases.

## OBJECTIVES

The student should be able to:
- Diagnose the common medical diseases.
- Manage the patients suffering from the common medical diseases.
- Prevent the common medical diseases.
- Discuss as to why pregnant women are prone to suffer from such diseases.
- List the causes of the medical diseases in pregnancy.

# URINARY TRACT INFECTION IN PREGNANCY

In general, urinary tract infection (U.T.I) is more common in females than in males because of the ease with which bacteria can gain access to the bladder through the short female urethra and the closeness of the urethra to the anus.

Pregnant women are more liable to U.T.I. than the non-pregnant ones because of the urinary stasis which is due to relaxation of the smooth muscles caused by progesterone. Progesterone also decreases peristaltic movements of the ureters. The enlarging uterus can also cause kinking of the ureters thus predisposing to development of hydro-ureters.

## Causative organisms of U.T.I

Urinary tract infection can be caused by:
- Escherichia coli. This is the commonest causative organism of U.T.I.
- Streptococcus faecalis.
- Pseudomonas aeroginosa.
- Klebsiella species.

The organisms usually ascend through the urinary tract thus causing urethritis, cystitis and pyelonephritis.

## Clinical features of U.T.1

Urinary tract infection during pregnancy can be symptomatic or asymptomatic.
- Symptomatic urinary tract infection. There are variable clinical features depending on the level of infection:
  - ➤ Dysuria that is painful micturation. Dysuria is common in urethritis and cystitis.

> ➢ Frequency, which is micturating more often. Usually the urine voided is in small amounts.
> ➢ Fever is common with pyelonephritis.
> ➢ Lower abdominal pains are common in cystitis and pyelonephritis.
> ➢ Tenderness in the renal angles indicates pyelonephritis.
> • Asymptomatic U.T.1.
> This is a laboratory diagnosis but patients do not have any of the above listed clinical features of U.T.1. Patients with asymptomatic U.T.1 are likely to develop symptomatic U.T.I. either during pregnancy or later in life.

> | URINE EXAMINATION SHOULD BE DONE ROUTENELY IN ALL PREGNANNT WOMEN. |
> | --- |

## Laboratory examinations

Urine examination is very important in all pregnant women. The urine should not be contaminated. The urine specimen can be one of the following:

> • Mid-stream urine. Mid-stream clean catch method is the one commonly used. To take this urine the patient should clean her vulva with normal saline, antiseptic should not be used. She discards the first portion of urine. She pours the middle portion of urine into a clean (or sterile if needed for culture) wide-mouthed bottle (or with the help of a funnel). She discards the third portion of urine.
> • Catheter specimen. The urethra is catheterised and the urine coming out through the catheter is taken for examination. This method of collecting urine is not recommended as catheterisation can cause urinary tract infection.
> • Suprapubic puncture urine sample.

The following investigations can be done to the urine collected:
- ➤ Microscopy.

  Microscopic examination of the urine is the first examination to be. Presence of pus cells or white cells (if there are more than 5 per high field) indicates urinary tract infection. Presence of red blood cells may mean involvement of renal parenchyma. Presence of casts and bacteria should also be looked for.
- ➤ Culture of the urine cannot be done at a health centre but a Clinical Officer is expected to interpret some of the culture results. Urine culture is done only if the urine looks infected, microscopically. The culture should be done immediately after the urine has been voided. If the culture cannot be done immediately, the urine can be kept at 4°C for a period of 24 hrs without being destroyed. After culture, colony counting is done. A count of:
  - ✓ $10^5$ or more colonies per ml of urine means the urine is infected.
  - ✓ $<10^3$ colonies means the urine was either contaminated or no infection.
  - ✓ Between $10^3$ and $10^4$ colonies means there is need to repeat the culture.

  It is only for the urine, which has significant colony count, that sensitivity test of the organisms is done.

Renal tests cannot be done at a health centre but a Clinical Officer should be able to interpret the results
- ➤ Blood urea.

  During pregnancy blood urea is 10–20 mg/dl while in non-pregnant women it is 20–40 mg/dl. An increase in blood urea indicates renal failure.

> ➢ Serum creatinine in pregnant and non-pregnant women is of the same, 1–2 mg/dl. A rise in serum creatinine indicates renal failure.

## Treatment of U.T.I

Both symptomatic and asymptomatic U.T.1. could be treated at a health centre, unless the patient is in severe pains or has developed complications. The treatment can be done at antenatal clinic. Patients who have significant abdominal pain need to be admitted in hospital and treatment started immediately as follows:

- Bed rest.
- Mild analgesics like acetylsalicylic acid tablets 2 tds for three days; unless the patient is in great pain, Pethidine injection is not necessary.
- The patient to drink a lot of water so as to improve urine flow.
- Urinary antiseptic like Nitrofurantoin 100mg tds for 7–10 days while waiting for the urine culture results.
- Antibiotics can be given according to sensitivity results. Use antibiotics that are not contraindicated during pregnancy. Many health centres in Tanzania are situated far from a hospital thus to send urine for culture might be difficult. In such situations wait for the outcome of the urinary antiseptic for about 48 hours, if there is no improvement in symptoms and/or urine microscopy still shows persistence of infections, switch to ampicillin or cloxacillin capsules 500 mg thrice a day for ten days. If still no improvement, refer patient to hospital.

## Complications of U.T.I

Complications of U.T.I can occur with either symptomatic or asymptomatic urinary tract infection.

- Recurrence of U.T.I. later in pregnancy or puerperium can occur, thus the importance of performing frequent urine microscopy. If recurrence is too often refer patient to hospital after delivery to rule out congenital malformations of urinary tract.
- Abortion.
- Preterm labour.
- Intrauterine foetal growth retardation.
- Intra-uterine foetal death.
- Anaemia. The anaemia is due to destruction of erythropoietin (produced by kidneys) which is an important enzyme for erythropoiesis.

# MALARIA IN PREGNANCY

Malaria is pan-endemic in many developing countries of the tropics. Pregnant women are more susceptible to malarial attacks than the non-pregnant. Pregnancy lowers immunity to malaria infection due to fall of antibodies. The factors leading to the fall in immunity during pregnancy include:
- Increased adreno-corticoid activity in pregnancy. Cortisone causes regression of lymphoid elements and reduces proliferation of macrophages. Steroids also increase parasitaemia.
- Pregnancy causes relative lymphocytosis.

## Complications of malaria in pregnancy

The complications of malaria in pregnancy include:
- Haemolytic anaemia. Anaemia is most marked in primigravidae due to their low immunity. The haemolysis due to Plasmodium falciparum infection is always in excess of the red blood cells destroyed by the parasites. The explanation of this excess haemolysis is that the infection causes hyperplasia of lymphoid tissues

and macrophages of reticulo-endothelial system, which in turn produce antibodies. The schizogony releases soluble antigen, which gets absorbed in red blood cells. The red blood cells, which have absorbed the antigen are phagocytosed by the macrophages and get haemolysed. Thus haemolysis can continue for about 24 hours after treatment of malaria in about 25% of patients. In about 5% of patients the haemolysis remains uncontrollable despite treatment unless prednisolone is given to the patient.

- Abortion is mainly due to high fever causing the uterus to contract.
- Preterm labour is also due to the fever.
- Intrauterine foetal growth retardation is common in primigravidae. The cause of the poor foetal growth rate is due to utero-placental insufficiency caused by the concentration of the parasites, lymphocytes and macrophages on the maternal surface of the placenta. Also there is a malarial toxin which retards foetal growth.
- Foetal distress.
- High stillbirth rate.
- Congenital malaria to the newborn is rare. The neonate is usually immune to malarial attacks because:
  ➤ Mosquitoes have selective feeding habits (mosquitoes prefer adult's blood).
  ➤ The baby's diet (breast milk) lacks para-aminobenzoic acid (PABA) which is required for development of plasmodia.
  ➤ Foetal haemoglobin may contribute to suppression of malaria infection.

## Investigation

The main investigation for malaria infection is blood slide. The blood slide can be thin film or thick film. The thick film is recommended for seeing of the parasites easily. In thin film it is not easy to see scanty infection but thin film is useful if typing of the plasmodium is needed. This investigation can be done at a health centre.

Modern antibody-antigen reaction agents are in the market. These are faster then the above method.

## Treatment of malaria in pregnancy

As mentioned complications of malaria can occur even in asymptomatic patients, all patients proved to have malaria parasites should be treated vigorously. The author performs routine blood slide check up for malaria parasites in all pregnant women.

The treatment of choice is chloroquine. In patients who are not vomiting, oral chloroquine is preferred. The regime is 600 mg (4 tabs) stat then repeated next day then 300 mg daily for three days; 4/4/ (2 x 3). If the patient is vomiting parentral chloroquine in the dose of either 200 mg intramuscularly for three days or 200 mg intramuscularly 8 hourly for 24 hours.

CHLOROQUINE DOES NOT CAUSE ABORTION OR PRETERM LABOUR.

An acetylsalicylic acid (Aspirin) or paracetamol tablet is given in the dose of 2 tablets thrice a day for three days so as to reduce the high temperature.

In chloroquine sensitive patients, comaquine can be given. In chloroquine-resistant malarial infection quinine can be given with caution, as it can cause abortion or preterm labour. It is not advisable for a Clinical Officer to prescribe quinine to his/her patients in a health centre, thus refer such patients to hospital.

## Prevention of malaria infection in pregnancy

As pregnant women have lowered immunity to malaria infection, they should be protected from malarial infection.

- Educate the pregnant women not to get mosquito bites by sleeping in mosquito nets and spraying their sleeping rooms with insecticides. Mosquito nets impregnated with mosquito repellents are available.
- The public should control mosquito-breeding places.
- Prophylaxis. Pregnant women should be given anti-malarial as said under antenatal care.

# DIABETES MELLITUS IN PREGNANCY

Diabetes mellitus is an endocrinological disease characterized by hyperglycaemia, polyuria and polyphagia. The main cause of diabetes mellitus is a relative lack of insulin. Pregnancy is a diabetogenic state. During pregnancy there are increased insulin antagonists like insulinase, corticosteroids, glucagon, growth hormone, adrenalin and human placental lactogen. The insulin antagonists cause increase in insulin production in normal pregnant women. Pregnancy can therefore worsen a diabetic condition or even put latent diabetes into picture.

During pregnancy normal fasting blood sugar should be 90–100 mg/dl while in the non-pregnant women blood sugar levels up to 120 mg/dl are normal. In pregnancy the renal threshold is lowered thus there is a high frequency of glycosuria (20% of women).

## Complications of diabetes mellitus in pregnancy

There are many complications of pregnancy that are due to diabetes mellitus, such as:

- Infertility. Infertility is common in diabetes. With the advent of insulin, about 20–30% of diabetics are fertile. The cause of infertility is not well known.
- Abortion. This is common in uncontrolled diabetes.
- High stillbirth rates.
- Intra-uterine foetal death commonly occurs in the last four (4) weeks of pregnancy, especially with the onset of diabetic keto-acidosis.
- Neonatal death. Early neonatal death is very high due to preterm deliveries and the babies born succumb to hypoglycaemia and infection easily.
- Urinary tract infection.
- Monilial infection is common, due to the high blood sugar levels.
- PIH is higher than in non-diabetics.
- Polyhydramnios is also common. The polyhydramnios is due to the diabetes mellitus itself or congenital foetal malformations which are common in diabetics.
- Respiratory distress syndrome (R.D.S.) is due to lung immaturity which complicates to atelectasis.
- Neonatal hypoglycaemia is common if feeding of the baby is delayed. The baby s born with high levels of insulin.
- The born babies are heavier than dates due to the effect of insulin (which causes body overgrowth) and deposition of fat. The baby is fat, bloated and oedematous. The baby is lethargic and can get cyanotic attacks easily.

## Classification of diabetes mellitus

Diabetes mellitus can be classified as follows:
- Potential diabetics are non-diabetics but have a greater chance of developing diabetes mellitus. Such patients are those with a positive family history of diabetes mellitus (like diabetic sibling, twin,

mother or father) or patients who had delivered a baby weighing 4.5 kg or more or those with recurrent and unexplained intra-uterine foetal deaths, stillbirths and early neonatal deaths.

- Latent diabetics are non-diabetics under normal conditions but become diabetics under stressful conditions like pregnancy, trauma. The patients usually return to normal when the stress is over.
- Gestational diabetics are the patients who develop diabetes mellitus during pregnancy and usually return to normal after delivery.
- Chemical diabetics are the patients who have no clinical features suggestive of diabetes mellitus but have an abnormal glucose tolerance test (G.T.T.).
- Clinical diabetics are the patients who have both clinical features of diabetes mellitus and an abnormal G.T.T.

## Investigation

Urine for sugar can be tested at a health centre using Klinistix. Any pregnant woman whose urine is found to contain sugar should have her fasting blood sugar tested by using Dextrostix. If sugar level is found to be greater than 110 mg/dl, transfer to hospital for glucose tolerance test.

TEST FOR URINE SUGAR ROUTENLY IN ALL PREGNANT WOMEN.

In the patient whose urine is positive for sugar, should also be tested for acetone using Acetest tablets. If the urine contains acetone or ketone bodies transfer such women to hospital.

## Management of a diabetic pregnant woman

The patient should immediately be referred to hospital where there is an obstetrician. The management of such a patient needs a combined effort of a physician, paediatrician and obstetrician. Patients are usually admitted in hospital for controlling the blood sugar and then can be treated as outpatients until delivery at 37 weeks of pregnancy.

- Insulin injection is the drug of choice. Many times the insulin dose needed is higher than in the non-pregnant. The insulin initiation is calculated as 0.7 i.u of insulin per kilogram body weight of the patient. Two thirds of the calculated dose is given in the morning as regular insulin and isophane (NPH) in the ratio of 1:2. The other one third of the calculated dose is given in the evening as regular insulin and NPH in the ratio of 1:1. This dose of insulin should be regulated according to the blood sugar levels.
- Oral hypoglycaemic like diabenese are contra-indicated in pregnancy because they are teratogenic, can cause neonatal hypoglycaemia and are slow acting.
- During treatment the blood sugar should be monitored closely 4–6 hourly. Monitoring of urine for control of blood sugar is not good as glycosuria is common during pregnancy without the patient being hyperglycaemic. Acetone and ketone bodies should be monitored closely.
- In well controlled patients pregnancy can go beyond 36 weeks of gestation but delivery is usually performed by the 37th week of gestation for fear of intra-uterine death. Vaginal delivery is recommended unless there are contra-indications to it like, history of previous caesarean section, malpresentation, failed induction or any other high risk factor. Trial of labour is not done in diabetics.

## Care of the newborn of a diabetic woman

The problems of the newborns are respiratory distress syndrome (R.D.S.), hypoglycaemia, hypocalcaemia, hyperbilirubinaemia, polycythemia and hypokalaemia. Therefore immediately after delivery:

- The baby's airway should be cleared by sucking its mucus.
- The baby should be kept warm, preferably in an incubator.
- The newborn should be fed with glucose solution as early as possible.
- The baby should be examined to rule out any congenital malformations.

Both the mother and her baby should be referred to hospital after resuscitation.

# ANAEMIA IN PREGNANCY

Anaemia is a common condition in pregnant women in Tanzania. In Bombo, Hospital, Tanga, about 37% of all antenatal admission is due to anaemia. By definition a woman is said to be anaemic if her haemoglobin level is less than 11.0gm/dl of blood.

## Causes of anaemia in pregnancy

There are many causes of anaemia in pregnancy:
- Haemodilution. During pregnancy the total blood volume increases by 40–50%. Plasma volume increases by 30–40% and the blood cells increase by 18–20%. This causes a relative haemodilution giving rise to "Physiological anaemia". In a well fed pregnant woman this physiological anaemia is not seen.
- Increased nutrient demand. During pregnancy there is an increased demand of nutrients to both mother and her foetus. Iron demand is increased by 1.0 gm (300 mg of iron is needed by the foetus while 700mg is needed by the mother). Folic acid demand is also increased. This is even more so in multiple pregnancy then in singleton pregnancies. It is also increased if pregnancies are repeated frequently.

- Deficiency of nutrients intake. The important nutrients commonly taken inadequate amounts are iron and folic acid. This is due to inadequate food intake. The food is taken inadequately either because of nausea, vomiting, distaste of food or poor foods (due to bad preparation as folic acid is heat labile). The food might just be not available; such foods as meat and fish in which iron is in abundance.
- Chronic blood loss. Women usually have lower haemoglobin compared to men due to their monthly blood loss, during menstruation. During pregnancy the woman is amenorrhoeic and saves about 250 mg of iron in the nine months of pregnancy. Chronic blood loss during pregnancy can occur in A.P.H., threatened abortion and hookworm infestation.
- Red cells destruction. Red cells have a life span of 120 days. They are destroyed in the liver and spleen. Red cells destruction is increased during malarial attacks or in sickle cell disease.

## Classification of anaemia in pregnancy

As in general medicine, anaemia in pregnancy can be classified as follows:
- Nutritional deficiency anaemia. The important nutrients for haemopoesis are iron, folic acid, vitamin B, vitamin C, thyroxin and proteins. Nutritional deficiency anaemia is the commonest type of anaemia during pregnancy. As said previously iron followed by folic acid deficiencies are common during pregnancy.
- Haemorrhagic anaemia. This type of anaemia in pregnancy can be caused by A.P.H., abortion and P.P.H.
- Haemolytic anaemia. The destruction of red cells in pregnancy could be due to malaria infection, urinary tract infection and sickle cell disease.

- Aplastic anaemia which is due to destruction of bone marrow can be due to lead poisoning. This type of anaemia is not common in pregnancy.

## Diagnosis of anaemia in pregnancy

- Clinically, an anaemic patient may complain of dizziness, palpitations and body weakness. On examination the patient will look pale.
- Investigations for anaemia include:
  ➢ Haemoglobin.
  ➢ Haematocrit.
  ➢ Stool examination for ova (mainly hookworm and ascaris ova).
  ➢ Blood slide for parasites.
  ➢ Urine for microscopy.
  ➢ Red cells morphology so as to know the type of anaemia. In iron deficiency anaemia the red blood cells will be microcytic and hypochromic; in folic acid or Vit.B deficiency anaemia the red cells will be macrocytic and normochromic; in haemolytic anaemia the red cells will be normocytic-normochromic but the reticulocyte count (number of immature red blood cells) will be higher than 1%.

## Iron deficiency anaemia in pregnancy

Iron deficiency anaemia is the most type of anaemia in pregnant women in third world countries. The main factors that give rise to iron deficiency anaemia include:

- Reduced iron intake due to excessive morning sickness or poor diet.
- Reduced iron absorption, especially if the woman takes more of insoluble iron compound. Magnesium trisilicate cheats iron thus

this drug should not be given simultaneously with iron tablets. Tea also reduces absorption of iron.
- Pregnancy creates an increased demand for iron more so in multiple pregnancy, multiparity, rapidly recurring pregnancies with delivery intervals of less than two years.
- Haemorrhage in present or previous pregnancies.

Treatment of iron deficiency anaemia depends on the gestation periods and severity of anaemia.

➢ If gestation period less than 34 weeks and haemoglobin is 9 gm/dl (60%) or above the patient can be treated at antenatal clinic with oral fersolate 200 mg thrice a day. The prescribed oral iron will increase haemoglobin by 1 gm per month of use. If the haemoglobin is less than 9 gm/dl but more than 6 gm/dl (40%) then the patient should be admitted and given parentral iron as described below. Parentral iron is also indicated if the patient has iron intolerance or malabsorption syndrome. The most common parentral iron given is imferon (IRON DEXTRAN). The other parentral iron is Jectofer.

The total imferon needed can be derived from:
✓ Manufacturer's table.
✓ Calculated by using the following formula.

$$0.66 \times \text{Body weight} \times \left(100 - \frac{\text{Hb} \times 100}{14.8}\right)$$

Where Body weight is in Kgms and Hb is haemoglobin of the patient in gm/dl.
This will give the total dose in grams. To get the dose in millilitres is to divide the answer above by 50. It is advisable to add 50 mg to the calculated dose for pregnant patients.

The calculated iron dose can be given by deep intra-muscular injection 2–5 mls on alternate days. So as not to stain the skin the intramuscular injection should be given in a Z-figure and the needle flushed with normal saline before withdrawing it from the muscles. Before administering the imferon a test for sensitivity to imferon should be done. The intramuscular injection can cause abscesses and is also suspected, though not proved, to be carcinogenic. The calculated dose can be given intravenously as a total dose (Total Dose Imferon T.D.I.). The calculated dose is diluted in 1000mls of 5% Dextrose or normal saline. Antihistamine like Promethazine 25 mg is given 30 minutes before starting the infusion. The infusion is started at 15 drops per minute and increased to 45 drops per minute if there is no reaction. No oral iron should be given after the infusion. Oral folic acid should be given as hidden folic acid deficiency may be unmasked.

**TID SHOULD BE GIVEN CAREFULLY AS IT IS NOT WITHOUT SIDE EFFECTS.**

The manufacturer's instruction should be followed carefully when giving T.D.I.

If the gestation period is 34 weeks or more such a patient should be transferred to hospital with donors for possible blood transfusion as she could deliver at any time and any blood loss might worsen the condition.

**ONE PINT OF BLOOD RAISES THE HAEMOGLODIN BY 1 GM/DL.**

> If the haemoglobin is 6 gm/dl or less such a patient has severe anaemia and should be referred to hospital immediately for blood transfusion regardless of the gestation period.

Due to the fear of transmission of Human Immunodeficiency Virus (HIV) the author is very conservative. If the woman is not in labour and has no symptoms of severe anaemia then imferon is given intramuscularly and advised to improve her diet; the patient should also be dewormed. If the patient is in labour 2–3 pints of blood (preferably packed cells) should be reserved. Labour should be managed actively. Blood transfusion could be started post-delivery. If the patient develops signs of congestive cardiac failure exchange blood transfusion can be life saving.

## Complications of anaemia during pregnancy

The complications of anaemia in pregnancy include:
- Infections. A pregnant woman who is anaemic is prone to urinary and genital tract infection during pregnancy and after delivery.
- Preterm labour.
- Intra-uterine foetal growth retardation due to inadequate nutrients.
- Intra-uterine death due to inadequate oxygen supply.
- Stillbirths.
- Increased perinatal mortality.
- Neonatal anaemia. The babies born have limited iron stores despite being born with normal haemoglobin.

## Prevention of anaemia during pregnancy

Some of the preventative measures include:
- Health education.

- Pregnant women should be advised to eat a balanced diet. Some of the traditional taboos like not eating eggs during pregnancy should be discouraged.
- Pregnant women should be advised to attend antenatal clinics early for early detection and treatment of anaemia.
- Prevention of malaria and hookworm should be a national priority.
- Prophylaxis against malaria and iron deficiency anaemia should be provided routinely as said under the chapter on antenatal care.
- Deworming. All patients found to have intestinal worms, especially hookworm, should be dewormed.

# CHAPTER 14

# INTRA-UTERINE FOETAL DEATH

## INTRODUCTION

The announcement of an intra-uterine foetal death is depressing to the mother. Thus the midwife should be 100% sure that the baby is dead in utero before revealing such a diagnosis to the mother.

## OBJECTIVES

The student should be able to:
- Define intra-uterine foetal death.
- List the causes of intra-uterine foetal death.
- List complications of intra-uterine foetal death.
- Diagnose intra-uterine foetal death.
- Manage a woman with a dead foetus at health centre.

## DEFINITION

Intra-uterine foetal death literally means the death of a foetus in utero. Intra-uterine foetal death includes death of the foetus before 12 weeks of gestation (missed abortion) and that which occurs later before delivery of the foetus. When the foetus is absorbed this is known as blighted ovum.

# CAUSES OF INTRA-UTERINE FOETAL DEATH

There are many causes of intra-uterine foetal death, such as:
- Maternal febrile illnesses due to any cause can kill the foetus directly. This is the commonest cause of intra-uterine foetal death in third world countries.
- PIH/eclampsia cause reduction of foetal oxygen supply thus the foetus dies due to asphyxia.
- Foetal malformations can causes death before, during or after labour; depending on the severity of the malformation.
- Cord accidents like cord prolapse; true cord knot or cord around the foetal neck can cause foetal death due to disturbance of foetal blood circulation.
- Placental insufficiency due to any cause.
- Diabetes mellitus.
- Renal conditions.
- A.B.O. and rhesus incompatibility.
- Post-maturity.
- Syphilis.

# DIAGNOSIS OF INTRA-UTERINE FOETAL DEATH

## Symptoms

The symptoms of intra-uterine foetal death include:
- Disappearance of symptoms of pregnancy.
- Patient not feeling foetal movements, if she had felt them earlier.
- Production of milk instead of colostrum.

- Vaginal brownish discharge. In such states, especially when the gestation period is less than 20 weeks and the pregnancy test positive, a diagnosis of threatened abortion is usually made.

## Signs

The signs for foetal death include:
- No foetal heart.
- The fundus may be stationary or smaller than dates or decreasing in height.
- The breasts, when expressed, will secrete milk instead of colostrum.

## Investigations

At the health centre a few investigations to prove foetal death can be performed.
- Urine for pregnancy test may be negative especially if the placenta is already dead. The pregnancy test may still be positive with a dead foetus if the test is done too early. Pregnancy test may be positive 2–4 weeks after death of the foetus or delivery.
- If radiological facilities are available then an abdominal X-ray can be taken two weeks after the suspected time of death. Taking the X-ray too early will not show many of the expected signs for foetal death. The X-ray can only be meaningful if taken after the gestation period of 16 weeks when the foetal skeleton is radiologically visible. The radiological signs include:
  - ➢ Accumulation of gas in the foetal heart and great vessels like the aorta and the vena cava.
  - ➢ Accumulation of gas between the foetal skull bones and the scalp giving the "holo sign".
  - ➢ Hyper-angulation of the foetal spine.
  - ➢ Narrowing of the inter-costal spaces.

> ➢ Crumbling of the foetus giving rise to "Ball's sign".
> ➢ Overlapping of the foetal skull sutures giving rise to "Spalding's sign.

Finding more than one of the listed features makes the radiological diagnosis.

- In centres with ultrasound machine, sonography should be done instead of X-ray. Ultrasound can diagnose foetal death earlier then before the symptoms and signs of IUFD. The foetal heart can be sonographically detected as early as seven weeks of pregnancy.

# COMPLICATIONS OF INTRA-UTERINE FOETAL DEATH (IUFD)

The complications of intra-uterine foetal death include:
- Hypofibrinogenaemia leading to bleeding tendency. This complication can occur in about 20% of foetus retained in utero for more than four weeks.
- Bacterial infections especially when the membranes have ruptured. A dead and macerated baby is good bacterial culture media.
- Psychological depression of the mother, husband and relatives at large.
- Maceration of the foetus. The dead baby undergoes a destructive aseptic process within 12–24 hours after the foetal death. The baby's skin becomes blackened and sloughs with ease.

MACERATED STILBIRTH NEARLY ALWAYS INDICATES THAT FOETAL DEATH DURING PREGNANCY AND NOT DURING LABOUR UNLESS THE LABOUR WAS SERIOUSLY PROLONGED.

- Postpartum haemorrhage due to hypofibrinogenaemia.

# TREATMENT OF IUFD

The patient should be referred to hospital. In hospital two types of management can be applied:

- Conservative management by waiting for spontaneous expulsion of the foetus. About 85% of the dead foetuses will be expelled spontaneously within 3–4 weeks of death. If the foetus is retained for more than four weeks attempts should be made to induce labour.
- Induction of labour can be done in anxious patients or those in whom the foetus is retained in utero for more than four. Medical induction is preferred.

ALWAYS GET READY FOR BLOOD TRANSFUSION IN CASE THE PATIENT DEVELOPS PPH.

- Surgical induction should not be done for fear of infection.
- Rarely caesarean section is indicated.

# CHAPTER 15

# NORMAL LABOUR

## INTRODUCTION

The climax of the care of a pregnant woman is at the time when she goes into labour. In the labour ward midwives are extremely busy and anxious as the ultimate goal of antenatal care is going to be proved during delivery. Labour is a stressful condition not only for the parturating mother but also for the midwives and relatives; all are anxiously awaiting the outcome of the labour. The Clinical Officer, as the chief midwife in his/her health centre, should be conversant with labour and delivery techniques.

## OBJECTIVES

The student should be able to:
- Define labour.
- Diagnose labour.
- Discuss briefly the mechanism of labour.
- Manage a woman in labour.

# DEFINITION OF LABOUR

Labour is a physiological process by which the foetus, placenta and membranes are expelled through the birth canal. The term 'labour' is used after the twenty fourth week of gestation, before then this process is called 'abortion.' Labour is said to be normal if it takes the normal expected period as described later. Labour is aptly named as there is considerable expenditure of energy during the first and second stages.

# DIAGNOSIS OF LABOUR

The diagnosis of labour can be done on a clinical basis.

- Lower abdominal pains. These pains are colicky in nature and radiating to the lower back. These pains are due to uterine contractions. Note that uterine contractions are present throughout pregnancy and become more frequent towards term. These contractions are called "Braxton Hick's contractions" or "false contractions". Braxton Hick's contractions are present before labour begins, especially in multiparous women. Braxton Hick's contractions can become painful enough to interfere with sleep, especially in the last weeks of pregnancy. These false contractions do not result in progressive labour. This is called" false labour".

> A SCREAMING WOMAN IS NOT NECESSARILY HAVING A UTERINE CONTRACTION.

True labour pains increase in intensity and decrease in interval as time goes. At the onset of true labour, pains come every 10–20 minutes and are fairly weak. The labour pains increase in strength, duration and frequency as labour progresses. The pains then come every 2–3 minutes and last for 30–90 seconds at the end of first stage. Uterine contractions can be palpated by the midwife abdominally.

- Progressive dilatation of the cervix. Cervical dilation can be diagnosed by pelvic examination. The midwife should note the degree of dilatation and effacement (shortening) of the cervix.
- Show. Show is the cervical plug which is formed during pregnancy. As the cervix dilates this cervical plug gets discharged. The show contains mucus mixed with blood.
- Descent of the presenting part. In women with high angle of inclination of the pelvis at times the foetal head delays to engage until late first stage.

True labour results in a progressive state of the above described clinical features. Labour is said to be progressing well and thus normal, if:

  ➢ The uterine contractions become stronger and regular as time passes.
  ➢ The cervix dilates progressively. The cervix should dilate at a minimum rate of 1 cm per hour in both multigravidae and primigravidae (in primgravidae 1.2 cm/hr while in multiparous is 1.5 cm/hr).
  ➢ The presenting part is descending into the pelvis.

# MECHANISM OF LABOUR

Mechanism of labour is a series of movements the foetus makes as it passes through the birth canal or the pelvis. The pelvis is a curved passage with different diameters at the inlet, mid cavity and outlet. The foetus has thus to adapt itself to the shape, size and curvature of the pelvis at different levels as it descends. To be able to manage labour properly the midwife should understand these foetal movements. While assisting a delivery, these foetal movements should be allowed to take place rather than being opposed. The following discussion of the mechanism of labour is applicable when the presenting part (i.e. the leading part) of the foetus is vertex.

- Descent of the foetus is the first foetal movement. In some women the foetal head descends into the pelvic brim and gets engaged that is the presenting diameter passes through the pelvic brim before onset of labour. In some women descent of the foetal head into the pelvis starts after onset of labour. In women with high angle of inclination of the pelvis at times the foetal head delays to engage until late first stage.

- Flexion of the foetus. The foetal head presents itself in the transverse diameter of the pelvic brim and the common position (that is the relationship of the denominator of the presenting part to the pelvis) being left occiput transverse (L.O.T). The right occiput transverse (R.O.T) is a normal position of the vertex too. As labour progresses the foetus becomes more flexed and the occipito-bregmatic diameter becomes the presenting diameter. When the presenting diameter has passed through the pelvic brim this is called "engagement". Engagement is a favourable sign indicating adequacy of the pelvis.

- Internal rotation. As labour continues and the foetal head descends into the mid cavity. It rotates from the L.O.T to left occiput anterior (LOA) or left occiput anterior (R.O.A.) if it was R.O.T before. The head is now lying on the oblique diameter of the pelvis and the neck twisted. The descent of the head continues and the vertex turns to occiput anterior (O.A.) as it reaches the pelvic floor marking the end of internal rotating. At the end of internal rotation the shoulders are in left or right oblique diameter of the pelvic brim.

- Extension of the head. As the occiput is below the symphysis, further descent of the foetus pushes the head forward and a larger segment of the presenting part becomes visible and "crowned" by the perineum. With further descent of the foetus and a movement of extension at the neck the occiput is delivered. Increased extension of the neck round the pubis delivers the bregma, brow and face of the foetal head. The shoulders by this time are lying obliquely in the mid cavity.

- Restitution. The head after being delivered spontaneously rotates to the position relative to the shoulders in the mid cavity. This movement is called restitution.
- External rotation. As descent of the foetus continues, the shoulders rotate to antero-posterior diameter of the pelvic outlet and the head follows the rotation of the shoulders so that the occiput comes to lie next to the mother's thigh. This movement of the head is called external rotation.
- Further descent and lateral flexion of the foetus causes the anterior shoulder of the foetus to pass under the pubic symphysis. The delivery of the anterior shoulder starts then the posterior shoulder follows then the whole body of the foetus is delivered.

# SOFT TISSUE CHANGES DURING LABOUR

The soft tissues involved are the uterus, cervix and the amniotic membranes.

- The uterine muscles contract and relax. During labour the uterine muscles contract but do not return to their former length during relaxation, thus as labour continues the muscles become shorter and thicker. This behaviour of uterine muscles is called "retraction". Retraction causes the uterine cavity to become progressively smaller thus pushing the foetus out. The area between the body of the uterus and the cervix is called the "isthmus". The isthmus contains mainly connective tissues and few muscles. The isthmus during uterine contractions continuously stretches and it does not retract. The isthmus becomes thin towards the end of labour and is called the lower segment.

- The formation of the lower segment causes shortening, thinning and taking up (i.e. being included into the lower segment) of the cervix. This is cervical effacement. The effacement and dilatation of the cervix continues until the cervix is flushed with the vaginal wall.
- Effacement and dilatation of the cervix leads to the separation of the amniotic membranes from the cervix thus allowing the formation of the fore waters. In the parous woman cervical dilatation and effacement usually occur together whereas in the primigravida effacement precedes cervical dilatation.

# THE STAGES OF LABOUR

Classically there are three stages of labour, though sometimes a fourth stage is described. These stages are:

- The first stage of labour is when regular uterine contraction start and ends when the cervix is fully dilated (10 cm diameter). In multigravidae patients this stage of labour lasts for about 8 hours while in primigravida patients this stage of labour can last up to 12 hours. It is divided into two phases:
  - ➤ Latent phase. This is from onset of labour until the cervix is 3 cm. dilated. This phase may take as long as 8hrs.
  - ➤ Active phase. This is from cervical dilatation of 3 cm (note that, in multiparous the cervix may be dilated while not in labour), until it is fully dilated. During this phase the cervix should dilate at least 1cm/hr. By simple mathematics, this phase should not last for more than 7hrs unless there is a problem.
- The second stage of labour starts when the cervix is fully dilated and ends when the baby is born. The second stage of labour lasts

for 15–30 minutes in multigravidae while in primigravida it can take 30–45 minutes. In the second stage uterine contractions become more frequent and powerful, the desire to bear down becomes strong and the woman experiences an urge to bear down.

- The third stage of labour starts immediately after the birth of the baby and ends after the expulsion of the placenta and its membranes. In both the multigravidae and the primigravidae the third stage takes 15 minutes to be completed.
- The fourth stage. This is the mechanical expulsion of the blood clots from the uterus after delivery of the placenta.

# MANAGEMENT OF LABOUR

Proper management of labour is essential. Many women will come to the health institution thinking that they are in labour. It is up to the midwife to prove that the woman is in true labour or not. The antenatal card should be checked so as to see any previously identified high risk factor(s).

- A detailed history is taken as outlined in the chapter on history taking. In particular checking for the onset of contractions, passage of show, leaking of liquor (indicating ruptured membranes) and any treatment given.
- A thorough examination should be performed as described under antenatal care; in particular abdominal examination of the pregnant uterus, cervical effacement and dilatation, presenting part, position and level of the presenting part.
- Cord prolapse or presentation should be ruled out. Note that the vaginal examination should be done aseptically.
- Blood pressure should be checked.
- Routine investigation includes:

> Urine for sugar, protein and acetone.
> Blood for haemoglobin and grouping and/or cross-matching in particular if the patient is anaemic.
- All high risk patients should be referred to hospital unless in late first stage.

## Management of first stage of labour

When the woman is proved to be in labour she is admitted to a labour ward. If she is in early first stage of labour and the membranes are not ruptured she should be given enema (so as to enhance labour and clear her rectum of faeces), and a hot bath. Then the membranes are ruptured. Rupturing of membranes (fore waters) helps to enhance labour, identify the colour of liquor and rule out cord prolapse.

The patient can be allowed to walk around the ward. She is allowed to take liquid diet with a lot of sugar for she will need the energy during the bearing down time. She should not be allowed to eat solid food. The following should be checked and recorded.
- Foetal heart rate should be monitored 1/2 hourly or more regularly if foetal distress is suspected. The normal foetal heart rate is 120–160 beats per minute. The foetal heart should be checked for its rate and character. The foetal heart should be monitored both while the uterus is relaxed and contracting. In centres with Cardiotocographic machine (CTG) it should be used instead of the Pinard stethoscope.
- Maternal blood pressure and pulse should be checked hourly.
- Uterine contractions should be checked hourly. While checking for the uterine contractions the level of the presenting head can be checked abdominally.
- Cervical dilation should be checked at least 4 hourly. The level and position of the presenting part to be checked vaginally, 4

hourly. During vaginal examination also check for the degree of moulding of the foetal skull bones. Moulding means overlapping of skull bones. The degree of moulding can be 1° when the bones just touch one another, 2° when the bones are overlapped but can be separated digitally and 3° when the bones are so much over-lapped that they cannot be separated digitally. Also check for caput succedaneum i.e. oedema of the scalp. Too frequent vaginal examinations increase the risk of infection even if done asceti-cally; thus during vaginal examination do all checks described above.

> **CERVICAL DILATATION SHOULD BE CHECKED AT LEAST FOUR HOURLY.**

- If the bladder is full the woman is encouraged to empty it. Unnecessary bladder catheterisation can cause urinary infection.

Bearing down efforts in first stage of labour will not enhance delivery of the baby but will only exhaust the mother and cause oedema of her cervix.

> **DISCORAGE THE WOMAN FROM BEARING DOWN DURING THE FIRST STAGE OF LABOUR.**

## Management of the second stage of labour

Once the cervix is fully dilated delivery of the baby should be expected at any time. The midwife should have prepared a delivery kit earlier. The woman lies on a delivery bed. The woman can deliver in the left lateral position, but usually the dorsal position is preferred. The mid-wife prepares himself/herself to assist the delivery.

A WOMAN IN SECOND STAGE OF LABOUR SHOULD NOT BE LEFT ALONE AT ANY ONE TIME.

During the second stage of labour uterine contractions become more frequent and powerful. The woman's desire to bear down becomes strong, but she should be discouraged from bearing down until the head has crowned. The technique of bearing down is the same as when passing hard stools. The bearing down is done during a uterine contraction. The woman should be instructed to breathe in and out fast in between contractions.

BEARING DOWN BEFORE THE FOETAL HEAD HAS CROWNED IS JUST GOING TO EXHAUST THE PATIENT.

The midwife starts to assist delivery when the head is seen in the vulva. The midwife scrubbed and wearing sterile gloves stands on the right side of the patient.

DELIVERY SHOULD BE CONDUCTED ASCEPTICALY.

- A sterile pad soaked in antiseptic is placed over the patient's gaping anus and some pressure is applied over the perineum until the occiput of the foetus has passed under the pubic symphysis. The perineal pressure helps to maintain flexion of the foetal head. The left hand of the midwife presses downwards on the most anterior part of the head of the foetus as it extends the vulva. This procedure also helps to maintain flexion of the head. The perineum should be watched at this stage for signs of impending tear so that episiotomy is done in time.
- When the head has been delivered, the baby's eyes and mouth are wiped. The head is let to restitute and do external rotation by itself. The midwife should check for cord around the head.

- The midwife then grasps the foetal head and directs it first towards the anus; pull it gently until the anterior shoulder is delivered. Then the head is pulled upwards towards the maternal pubic symphysis to deliver the posterior shoulder. The posterior shoulder should be delivered carefully as there is still the risk of tearing the perineum during this stage.
- Then the midwife grasps the delivered shoulders; the trunk and legs of the foetus are delivered by lifting the baby up over the maternal pubis. The baby's mouth and nose are drained by posture or suction.
- The born baby is then laid between the mother's legs and the cord ligated and divided when it stops pulsating. The baby is then handed to an assistant for resuscitation (see chapter on care of the newborn).

A WOMAN IN LABOUR SHOULD NOT BE LEFT ALONE UNTIL THE PLACENTA HAS BEEN DELIVERED COMPLETELY.

## Management of the third stage of labour

There are two methods of delivering the placenta, either passive or active.

- The passive method of delivering the placenta is the one in which oxytocics are not used. This method is indicated in patients with cardiac or hypertensive diseases; if a student is being supervised to deliver the placenta passively or if twins are diagnosed or suspected, the oxytocics are delayed until the delivery of all the babies. After handing the born baby to an assistant the midwife:
  ➢ Puts a bowl against the perineum to collect the blood.
  ➢ Puts his/her hand still on the fundus, fondling the fundus or even rubbing it, is contraindicated as it may cause partial separation of the placenta leading to P.P.H.

> **IT IS DANGEROUS TO FONDLE THE UTERUS BEFORE THE PLACENTA IS COMPLETELY DELIVERED.**

- ➤ Signs of spontaneous separation of placenta are waited for. The signs include:
  - ✓ The uterus becoming hard and rising.
  - ✓ The cord lengthening.
  - ✓ Some vaginal bleeding.
  - ✓ The patient may get abdominal pain due to uterine contraction.
- ➤ After the signs of placental separation have taken place the patient is asked to bear down or the midwife applies gentle fundal pressure.
- ➤ While the placenta is being delivered it is held with both hands, by the midwife, and gently rotated so as to allow the membranes to slowly peal off.
- ➤ After complete delivery of the placenta the fundus of the uterus is rubbed to stimulate a contraction. The uterus is also squeezed so as to expel any blood clots.

> **FAILURE TO EXPEL BLOOD CLOTS FROM THE UTERUS WILL LEAD TO PPH.**

- ➤ The vagina, labia and perineum are then checked for tears and other injuries and repaired. The vulva is swabbed clean and a sterile pad is placed over the vagina to collect lochia.
- ➤ The placenta and membranes are examined to detect any deficiencies, diseases or retained parts. If any part of the placenta is suspected to be missing then the uterine cavity should immediately be explored manually.

> The blood collected in the bowl is measured and recorded. The patient should be observed in the labour ward for at least one hour as vaginal bleeding may start at any time.

> When all is well the patient is transferred to the postnatal ward to rest.

• Active management of the third stage involves the use of oxytocics. The oxytocic commonly used is ergometrine 0.5 mg. Ergometrine when given intramuscularly acts within 5–7 minutes while if given intravenously it acts within 45 seconds. Syntometrine is also used. Syntometrine acts on the fundus and lower segment while ergometrine acts mostly on the fundus.

> Use of oxytocics during third stage reduces P.P.H. greatly and enhances delivery of the placenta. Use of oxytocics is thus, especially, a must in patients who are at risk of P.P.H. (see chapter under P.P.H.). In the patients who are at high risk of developing P.P.H, intravenous ergometrine is preferred. Ergometrine should not be used in patients with heart diseases or hypertension and in multiple pregnancy when all the babies are not delivered.

> Oxytocics can be given at different stages of labour.

   ✓ After crowning of the foetal head. Giving oxytocics at crowning achieves maximum prevention of P.P.H. but may lead to death of an undiagnosed twin and is dangerous if shoulder obstruction at the pelvic outlet occurs.

   ✓ After delivery of the anterior shoulder. This will prevent P.P.H. in most cases. This is the best stage to give oxytocics in routine deliveries.

   ✓ After the birth of the baby. P.P.H. may occur before the drug acts.

   ✓ After delivery of the placenta. At this stage a number of patients will have had P.P.H. though the danger of missing an undiagnosed twin is nil.

Routinely the third stage of labour is managed actively with controlled cord traction (Brandt-Andrews Method):

➤ Ergometrine is given intramuscularly after the delivery of the anterior shoulder.

➤ After the baby is born and handed to an assistant a uterine contraction is awaited and then the cord is held firmly with the right hand and gently pulled. The left hand holds the uterus above the symphysis pubis. The cord is first pulled downwards and then upwards as the placenta is being delivered. This is called controlled cord traction.

➤ The placenta is held and managed as under passive methods.

# CHAPTER 16

# INDUCTION OF LABOUR

## INTRODUCTION

Induction of labour is the process of artificial stimulation of labour. Induction of labour is a very common procedure in many labour wards world wide.

## OBJECTIVES

It is expected that at the end of this chapter the student will be able to:
- Define induction of labour.
- List the indications of induction.
- List the different methods of induction.
- List the contra-indications and complications of each method of induction of labour.
- Perform induction of labour safely.

## DEFINITION

See under introduction.

# INDICATIONS OF INDUCTION OF LABOUR

There are maternal and foetal indications of induction of labour.
- Foetal indications include.
  There are three main foetal indications for induction of labour.
  - Intra-uterine foetal growth retardation (I.U.F.G.R.).
  - Intra-uterine foetal death (I.U.F.D).
  - Haemolytic diseases of the foetus as in Rhesus incompatibility.
- Maternal indications include.
  There are many maternal indications. These include:
  - Placental-insufficiency (due to PIH/eclampsia).
  - Postmaturity.
  - Antepartum haemorrhage.
  - Diabetes mellitus.
  - Hypertensive illness in pregnancy.
  - Premature rupture of membranes (PROM).

# METHODS OF INDUCTION

There are two major methods of induction of labour, medical and surgical.
- Surgical indication of labour
  There are two main types of surgical induction of labour:
  - Membrane sweeping.
    Membrane sweeping means detaching the amniotic membrane of the fore waters from the lower segment of the uterus. Membrane sweeping is done by pushing a finger between the amniotic membranes and the uterus and rotate the finger through 360°. Membrane sweeping can start a "Ferguson's reflex" which in turn can cause release of oxytocin and

prostaglandin, which stimulate the uterus and make it contract.

➤ Amniotomy.

Amniotomy is the artificial rupturing of membranes. The membranes can either be the bag of hind-waters or fore-waters. Amniotomy of the bag of fore waters is the one commonly used.

## Medical Induction of labour

There are three main ways of medical induction.

- Bowel stimulation.

  Bowel stimulation causes a "Ferguson's reflex" to the uterus. Bowel stimulation can be done by either giving an enema or a purgative. Historically a woman in labour was given oil (castor oil as a purgative), enema and hot bath, thus the term O.B.E. was usually in the order of O.E.B.

- Oxytocics are also used for induction. In the past, extracts of animal pituitary glands were used but now a synthetic oxytocic known as Syntocinon is used. The Syntocinon is given intravenously as the oral route is ineffective and the intramuscular route is dangerous in case of over dosage.

- Prostaglandins are new drugs, which are more effective than oxytocics. Mesoprostal (Cytotec) which is a synthetic Prostaglandin $E_1$ ($PGE_1$) analogue is common in many developing countries. Mifepristone (RU-486) is common in developed countries.

# COMPLICATIONS OF INDUCTION OF LABOUR

None of the mentioned methods of induction of labour is free from complications.

# Surgical Induction

- Amniotomy has more complications than membrane sweeping; though amniotomy is more effective than membrane sweeping. Most of the following complications are for amniotomy.
  - ➢ Failure to start labour. In a successful amniotomy, labour starts within six hours. Amniotomy is more successful in women of high parity, advanced pregnancy and when the cervix is ripe and the presenting part is low in the pelvis.
  - ➢ Infection of the liquor and amniotic membrane (amnionitis) is evident if the amniotomy is not done aseptically or if labour is prolonged for more than 24 hours.

> SURGICAL INDUCTION COMMITS THE MIDWIFE TO DELIVER HER/HIS PATIENT WITHIN 24 HOURS.

  - ➢ Cord prolapse. Cord prolapse is a common complication in the rupture of fore-waters, especially if the presenting part is high or ill-fitting to the pelvic brim; or if the amniotic fluid is allowed to drain out suddenly or if there is already a cord presentation.

> RULE OUT CORD PROLAPSE WHEN THE FORE WATERS HAVE RUPTURED WHETHER ARTIFICIALLY OR SPONTENOUSLY.

  - ➢ Abruptio placenta. Abruptio placenta can occur if the amniotic fluid is released suddenly.
  - ➢ Preterm. The baby can be born preterm if induction is done before 37 weeks gestation. The delivery of the preterm baby can be done intentionally as in diabetic mothers or accidentally due to wrong dates when other facilities of estimating age of foetus are not available.

> ➢ Other rare complications include bleeding from the mother or the baby (especially when performing amniotomy of hind waters) and pulmonary embolism of the amniotic fluid.

## Medical Induction

Complications due to medical induction of labour are mainly for oxytocin or prostaglandin.

- Failure to start labour. The factors, which influence the success of amniotomy, hold true for use of oxytocin or prostaglandin.
- Over-infusion. Over loading the cardiovascular system can occur in the drip method of administering oxytocin.
- Foetal distress.
- Tetanic spasms of the uterus. The uterus can go into tetanic spasms if induction is done in a grand multiparous woman, the concentration is too high or if the drug is given too rapidly.
- Rupture of uterus. Rupture of uterus is unlikely to occur in the primigravida. The uterus can easily rupture if induction is done in multiparous women and in women with previous caesarean section scar.

> OXYTOCICS/PROSTAGLANDINS ARE GOOD INDUCERS OF LABOUR WHEN USED CAREFULLY OTHERWISE THEY CAN BE VERY DANGEROUS.

# CONTRAINDICATIONS TO INDUCTION OF LABOUR

Each of the previously mentioned methods of induction of labour has its own contraindications. The following is a discussion of the contraindications.

## Surgical induction

There are only a few contra-indications to surgical induction.
- Intra-uterine foetal death, for fear of introducing infection.
- Presence of infection in the vagina or vulva.
- Presence of diarrhoea, especially for amniotomy for fear of infection.
- Abnormal lie or malpresentation.

## Medical induction

Contra-indications to medical induction are more for use of oxytocin and prostaglandins.
- Diarrhoea. This is a contraindication for bowel stimulation as the drugs used can worsen the diarrhoea.
- High parity. Rupture of uterus is possible in the grand multiparous women.
- Previous caesarean section. The uterus can rupture with ease.
- Cephalo-pelvic disproportion.

# COMMON REGIME OF INDUCTION OF LABOUR

Each of the methods of induction of labour discussed earlier can induce labour on its own. Using a combination of the above methods of induction increases the success rate. It is common to combine surgical and medical methods of induction. The following is the schedule of induction in a woman with no contraindication to the methods.
- Enema. Enema is given the night before administering Syntocinon/prostaglandin. The author prefers to give enema for two consecutive evenings up to the night before starting

Syntocinon. Some patients will go into labour before the next step.

- Medical induction.
    - ➤ Syntocinon drip. On the following morning the patient is given a warm bath and asked to empty her bladder and rectum. A Syntocinon drip is set early in the morning at around 7–8 am. Five international units (10 i.u) diluted in 1000 mls of 5% Dextrose (10 Um/ml.) The drip is started at 20 drops per minute and the rate is increased by 10 drops after 30 minutes to maximum of 60 drops per min. depending on the uterine contractions. If the diluted drip is finished and the uterine contractions are not satisfactory higher concentration of syntocinon can be made but not to exceed 10 i.u in 1000 mls of 5% Dextrose. The same escalating speed of the drip is done. If uterine contractions are satisfactory the same concentration and rate of the Syntocinon drip are maintained.

In a centre with infusion pump then the syntocinon can be administered as shown in the table below.

## Oxytocin Infusion Table

| Infusion rate (mls/hr) | Dose of Oxytocin (mU/min) |
|---|---|
| 15 | 2.5 |
| 30 | 5 |
| 60 | 10 |
| 120 | 20 |
| 180 | 30 |
| 240 | 40 |

Smaller doses of syntocinon like 2.5units or 5 units may be used per litre. The infusion rate is increased until an active contraction pattern is established (1 contraction every 3 minutes). Once this is achieved, the infusion rate is maintained at this dose.

> ➤ Cytotec seems to be overtaking syntocinon. It is administered vaginally, deep into the posterior fornix, 50–100 µg stat. The dose can be repeated after eight hours if no uterine contractions.

- Amniotomy. Rupture of the bag of fore-waters by using Kocher forceps is preformed immediately after starting Syntocinon drip. It is the author's observation that delaying this procedure delays contraction and thus prolongs the induction-delivery interval. Amniotomy should not be done if cytotec is used for induction as the draining liquor will drain the tablet out.

---

**PATIENTS SHOULD BE INDUCED IN THE MORNING.**

---

# CHAPTER 17

# OPERATIVE DELIVERY

## INTRODUCTION

Obstetric operative deliveries are common procedures in many labour wards. There are many procedures, but all can be classified into two groups, those meant to facilitate vaginal delivery and those meant to by-pass vaginal delivery. This chapter will consider in detail the operative procedures that a Clinical Officer is expected to be able to do and those, which he/she can't do, will be described briefly.

## OBJECTIVES

The student should be able to:
- Define operative delivery.
- List five operative deliveries.
- List the indications and conditions for performing artificial rupture of membranes, episiotomy, vacuum extraction, symphysiotomy, caesarean section and forceps deliveries.
- Perform artificial rupture of membranes, episiotomy and vacuum extraction.

# DEFINITION

Operative delivery means any surgical obstetric procedure, which is done to effect delivery of the foetus.

# ARTIFICIAL RUPTURE OF MEMBRANES (A.R.M)

Artificial rupture of membrane is the commonest and oldest operative delivery. Anyone practising midwifery should have skills of A.R.M. As described under induction of labour the rupture of fore-waters is much preferred, thus the following discussion will be limited to this method.

## Technique of performing A.R.M

Artificial rupture of membranes should be performed aseptically. The procedure is usually without anaesthesia or sedatives.

- The patient is placed in dorsal position, with her legs flexed and abducted.
- The midwife scrubs and wears sterile gloves, usually on the right hand, and swabs the vulva with antiseptic.
- The midwife inserts his/her fingers (the first and middle fingers) of the gloved hand into the vagina and through the cervical canal until membranes are felt.
- The membranes are swept from the lower uterine segment.
- A sterile Kocher forceps is picked using the ungloved hand and introduced into the vagina.
- After reaching the membranes, the Kocher is used to tear the membranes while the gloved hand is in the vagina. Then the amniotic liquor is let out slowly.
- After ruling out cord prolapse the vaginal hand is removed. If the presenting part is high an assistant can push it into the pelvic brim, abdominally, before A.R.M.

## Indications of A.R.M

The main indication of A.R.M. is induction or augmentation of labour. Other advantages of A.R.M. include seeing the colour of liquor and preventing cord prolapse.

## Contraindications to A.R.M

- Abnormal lie of the foetus.
  - ➤ Transverse lie.
  - ➤ Oblique lie.
- Abnormal presentation.
  - ➤ Breech.
  - ➤ Shoulder.
- Infection in the vagina.
- Multiple pregnancy.
- Pre-term pregnancy.
- Diarrhoea.

## Dangers of A.R.M

Refer to chapter on Induction of Labour.

## Management of patient after A.R.M

Refer to chapter on Induction of Labour.

# EPISIOTOMY

Episiotomy is the next commonest operative procedure in labour wards worldwide. Episiotomy means deliberate incision of the perineum with an aim of increasing the vaginal diameter.

# Advantages of episiotomy

- Ensures an easier and quicker and therefore safe delivery of the foetus.
- Prevents injury to the maternal soft tissues.
- Prevents laceration of the perineum.

> A GENEROUS EPISIOTOMY IS EASIER TO REPAIR THAN A PERINEAL TEAR.

# Indications of episiotomy

- Impending perineal tear or the perineum is tearing.
- Foetal distress in second stage.
- Delivery of preterm baby.
- Rigid perineum.
- Breech delivery.
- Vacuum extraction or forceps delivery.
- Symphysiotomy.
- Destructive operation.

# Types of episiotomies (see fig.–15)

- Midline incision through the fourchette and perineal body. This type of episiotomy has the advantage that no blood vessels are encountered and the repair is simple. If this type of episiotomy extends it may involve the anal sphincter or the rectum.
- Lateral incision. This causes troublesome bleeding and damages the Bartholin's gland. It does not widen the vagina appreciably; thus it is no longer done.
- Postero-lateral incision is the most commonly done.
- J-shaped is a theoretical compromise incision, which becomes a postero-lateral incision.

## Technique of performing episiotomy

In a conscious patient the episiotomy should be done under local anaesthesia. It is not true that a woman does not feel pain at the height of uterine contraction. Episiotomy should be done aseptically with the midwife wearing sterile gloves on both hands.

- The patient is put either in lithotomy position or dorsal position with both legs flexed and abducted.
- The perineum is swabbed with antiseptic.
- 8–10 mls of 1% Lignocaine is infiltrated around the perineum in a triangular shape with apex at the fourchette. The skin and deeper muscles should also be infiltrated.
- Middle and index fingers of the left hand are inserted into the vagina and the perineum stretched. A generous episiotomy is performed using a big and sharp episiotomy scissors. Any significant bleeding blood vessel should be clamped with an artery forceps.

## Repair of episiotomy

The repair of episiotomy should be done immediately after delivery of the placenta as the lignocaine is still working. Delay in the repair of episiotomy may cause P.P.H. and/or allow the incision to be infected.

- Before repairing the episiotomy the vagina should be inspected any other tears.
- A gauze swab is inserted high deep into the vagina so that the apex is well visualized. The vaginal gauze will soak any bleeding from the uterus thus making the operation site dry.
- The author prefers to use catgut No.0. Starting from above the apex, with a round-bodied needle, a knot is tied and then a continuous suture is done to stitch the vaginal wall. The continuous suture ends just below the hymen. Then the perineal muscles and skin are sutured separately with interrupted catgut whose knots are buried.

- Then the vaginal gauze is removed after, checking that haemostasis has been maintained at the episiotomy site.
- A finger is inserted into the rectum to make sure that the rectum has not been sutured.

## Care of patient after repair of episiotomy

Usually if the sutures are not too tight the patient will not complain of vulval pain. As the vulva is well vascularised no antibiotics are needed. The patient can start walking as soon as she wishes. She can have normal puerperal care but she should not use hot water for vulval toilet. Hot water will make the sutures weak and break. Usually the sutures will be absorbed. The bowels are not confined.

A patient who had a previous episiotomy will not necessarily have another episiotomy in subsequent pregnancies unless otherwise indicated.

# SYMPHYSIOTOMY

Symphysiotomy is a procedure, which is losing its popularity. The author does not prefer the procedure but there are still some obstetricians who are fond of it. The Clinical Officer is not supposed to perform this procedure. Symphysiotomy essentially involves the cutting of the pubic symphysis through its fibro-cartilaginous tissue joining the two bones.

## Complications of symphysiotomy

In inexperienced hands and poor nursing care symphysiotomy can have the following complications:
- Haematoma over the mons pubis.

- Urethro-vaginal or vesico-vaginal fistula leading to urinary incontinence.
- Wobbling gait due to separation of the pubic bones.
- Chronic pain at the pubic bones.

## Care of patient after symphysiotomy

After symphysiotomy the patient needs good nursing care.
- Usually no prophylactic antibiotics needed.
- An indwelling and continuous draining urinary catheter should be inserted into the bladder for at least 48 hours.
- The patient should be nursed on her sides for at least three days. During this period she should not be allowed to lie on dorsal position at anyone time. When turning of the patient, her legs should be held together, but there is no need of tying them together.

# VACUUM EXTRACTION

Vacuum extractor (ventouse) (fig.–16) is an instrument that applies traction onto the foetal head by means of a suction cup attached to the scalp. The vacuum extractor is a substitute for the obstetric forceps.

## Types of vacuum extraction

There are two types of vacuum extraction, depending on the level of the presenting head.
- Low cavity vacuum extraction (L.C.V.E). If the foetal skull bones are below the ischial spines.
- High cavity vacuum extraction (H.C.V.E.). If the foetal skull bones are above the ischial spines.

The preferred vacuum extraction is the LCVE. The HCVE is not recommended due to its complications. The only indication for HCVE is in retained second twin and prolapse of cord.

## Prerequisites for vacuum extraction (V.E)

Before applying the vacuum the patient should be examined fully to make sure that:
- The foetus presents by the vertex and not by any other presentation. Malposition of the vertex is not a contraindication.
- The pelvis must be adequate for the foetus. The vacuum extractor cannot overcome cephalo-pelvic disproportion.
- The cervix is fully dilated.
- There must be good uterine contraction and maternal co-operation.

## Technique of V.E

The tubes, vacuum cup and traction plate should be pre-sterilized. The instrument is assembled as in fig.–16.
- The patient should have an empty bladder or is catheterised.
- The patient is put in lithotomy position with her legs supported on stirrups.
- The attendant well scrubbed and wears sterile gloves; cleans the vulva with antiseptic and performs a pelvic assessment to rule out cephalo-pelvic disproportion and also determines the presentation and position of the foetus. The level of the presenting part is also determined.
- The perineum is infiltrated with 1% lignocaine and episiotomy performed as usual. The largest cup of the extractor available (size 5 or 6) is lubricated and introduced into the vagina and applied to the foetal head as low as possible. Vaginal tissues are checked so that they are not included in the cup.

- An assistant closes the pressure screw of the extractor and pumps the extractor slowly until pressure on the gauge is 0.2 kg/sq.cm. The attendant checks around the cup to make sure that no vaginal tissue or the cervix is trapped in the cup. The assistant further pumps the extractor slowly at the pressure of 0.2 kg/sq.cm. every two minutes until the gauge reads 0.8kg/sq.cm. This pressure thus created gives the cup good grip on the foetal scalp. The attendant applies a steady and continuous on the tube following the sacral curvature.

## Functions of the V. E

- The main function of the vacuum extractor is to assist the uterine contractions and the maternal bearing down efforts in delivering of the head.
- A secondary function is to rotate the foetal head.

## Indications for V. E

Vacuum extraction can be used in:
- Delayed second stage.
- Second stage, in conditions where the woman is not supposed to bear down during delivery; such as in maternal distress, cardiac diseases, bronchi asthma, PIH, pulmonary tuberculosis and an exhausted woman.
- Prolapse of the cord in second stage.
- Foetal distress in second stage; if the procedure is not going to take long.

## Indications for discontinuing V. E

There is no point in attempting trial of vacuum. V.E. should be stopped if:
- Delivery is not completed within 15 minutes of traction.

- The cup slips off three times. This shows that there could be an undiagnosed disproportion.
- There is no delivery after three sustained pulls with contractions.

## Complications of V.E

Vacuum extraction is a safe procedure if done properly otherwise the following complications can arise:
- Tear of the vagina and/or cervix.
- Chignon. This is an artificial caput made by the suction force of the cup on the foetal scalp. This is normal oedema of the scalp, which usually subsides spontaneously within 12–60 hours.
- Scalp haematoma and sloughing of the scalp is due to excessive traction and/or pressure.

# CAESAREAN SECTION

Caesarean section means the removal of the foetus from an intact uterus by abdominal operation. Caesarean section is a procedure that a Clinical Officer/Midwife should not attempt to do but he/she is expected to know the indications, complications and the management of a pregnant woman who had undergone a previous caesarean section.

# CAESAREAN SECTION

Caesarean section means the removal of the foetus from an intact uterus by abdominal operation. Caesarean section is a procedure that a Clinical Officer/Midwife should not attempt to do but he/she is expected to know the indications, complications and the management of a pregnant woman who had undergone a previous caesarean section.

## Types of caesarean section

There are two main types of caesarean section, see fig.–17.

- The lower segment Caesarean Section (LSCS). This is the one commonly recommended and done. This type of caesarean has many advantages.
  - ➢ Bleeds less than classical caesarean section.
  - ➢ Heals better than classical caesarean section.
  - ➢ Less chances of infection than classical caesarean section.
  - ➢ A woman who had undergone LSCS can be given trial of scar.
  - ➢ LSCS has less chances of spontaneous rupture later than classical section.

  The LSCS is done by incising the uterus transversely on the anterior aspect of the lower segment.

- The classical caesarean section is the incision of the uterus longitudinally on the anterior aspect of the upper segment. This type of caesarean section is not preferred.
  - ➢ Bleeds more than LSCS.
  - ➢ Heals poorly than LSCS.
  - ➢ Higher chances of getting infected than LSCS.
  - ➢ Ruptures easily during pregnancy and/or labour, thus it is recommended that bilateral tubal ligation should be done if this type of operation is performed. The only indications for classical caesarean section are:
    - ✓ Impacted shoulder of the foetus.
    - ✓ Dense adhesions in the lower segment.
    - ✓ Mother is dead.
    - ✓ Hydrocephalus foetus.

# Indications for Caesarean section

Caesarean section is performed so as to save the life of the mother and or the foetus.

- Foetal indications for caesarean section include.
  - ➢ Foetal distress. This is the commonest indication.
  - ➢ Cord prolapse.
  - ➢ Transverse lie.
  - ➢ Big baby.
  - ➢ Foetal malpresentation like impacted shoulder, brow and face presentation.
  - ➢ Breech presentation especially in primigravidae.
  - ➢ Deep Transverse Arrest of foetal head.
  - ➢ Undescending foetal head.
  - ➢ Persistent occiput posterior during labour.
- Maternal indications for caesarean section include.
  - ➢ Cephalo-pelvic disproportion (CPD). This is the commonest indication.
  - ➢ Obstructed labour.
  - ➢ Previous two caesarean sections.
  - ➢ A.P .H. of major degree.
  - ➢ Severe PIH/Eclampsia.
  - ➢ Elderly primigravida with cephalo-pelvic disproportion.
  - ➢ Failed trial of labour.

Caesarean section (C/S) can be either elective or emergency.

  - ➢ Elective caesarean. This is a planned C/S. It is usually done at the end of the pregnancy (usually done 10–14 days before E.D.D.). Some of the indications for elective caesarean section include:
    - ✓ Two or more previous caesarean sections.

✓ Breech in primigravidae, borderline pelvis or with other high risk factors.
✓ Abnormal lie like transverse and oblique lie.

Clinical Officer/Midwife is supposed to detect such indications and refer the patient to hospital around 36–38 weeks of gestation, for caesarean section. During pregnancy the Clinical Officer should make sure that patients have good haemoglobin. Advise donors to be within reach for donating blood to the patient for the operation.

➢ Emergency caesarean section. This is an unplanned C/S which is performed as an emergency procedure. In such a patient, vaginal delivery had been anticipated but unfortunately something went wrong with the foetus or the woman, during pregnancy or labour, which dictates an emergence C/S (see indications for caesarean section). The patient should be referred to hospital immediately. A trained midwife and relatives escort the patient.

## Complications of caesarean section

The main complications of caesarean section include:
- Haemorrhage during and after operation.
- Anaesthetic accidents like anaesthetic shock, Mendelson's syndrome (aspiration of gastric contents during anaesthesia).
- Infection.
- Peritoneal adhesions.
- In subsequent pregnancy and/or labour a scarred uterus can rupture.

## Management of patient with previous caesarean section

- During pregnancy. These can be managed at Health centre antenatal clinic. During antenatal period the patient, should have good haemoglobin and her blood group and Rhesus factor should be known. The patient should be referred and admitted to hospital at around 36–38 weeks of gestation for delivery .The patient could be delivered either vaginally or by caesarean section.

- Trial of vaginal delivery is done when it has been decided to try the scar (trial of scar). Pre-requisites for trial of scar include:
  - ➢ The uterus should be sound that is no suspicion of the scar being weak.
  - ➢ There should be no malpresentation or malposition.
  - ➢ The trial should be done in hospital equipped for performing emergency caesarean section.

> TRIAL OF SCAR SHOULD NOT BE ATTEMPTED IN A HEALTH CENTRE.

In a successful trial of scar check the integrity of the uterine scar immediately after delivery of the placenta. The patient should be observed for 48 hours in the postnatal ward. Monitor pulse, blood pressure, temperature and watch and report to doctor any excessive vaginal bleeding. Trial of scar is said to have failed if there are signs and symptoms of impending uterine rupture, which including:

- ✓ Tenderness over uterine scar.
- ✓ Vaginal bleeding.
- ✓ Foetal distress.
- ✓ Maternal pulse increasing and or blood pressure decreasing.
- ✓ Labour not progressing well.

In failed trial of scar emergency caesarean section should be done.

## Indications for elective caesarean section in a patient with previous caesarean section include

- Two or more previous caesarean section. Allowing such a patient to deliver vaginally is gross mismanagement.

A WOMAN WHO HAD CAESAREAN SECTION TWICE SHOULD ALWAYS BE DELIVERED BY CAESAREAN SECTION.

- Previous history of ruptured uterus. Such patients should have been sterilized during the previous laparotomy.
- Previous classical caesarean section. Such patients should have been sterilized during the previous operation.
- Others as for the contraindication for trial of scar.

# OTHER OPERATIVE DELIVERIES

These other operative deliveries will be mentioned just to complete the list.

- Forceps delivery. Its indications are more or less as those for vacuum extraction. Forceps delivery should not be done by a Clinical Officer/Midwife.
- Destructive operation. This means destroying the baby or cutting the foetus into pieces (embryotomy). This procedure is done to a dead baby. The baby is cut so that it can be delivered vaginally. Such operations include:
  - ➢ Craniotomy (perforating the foetal head).
  - ➢ Decapitation (cutting the foetal neck).
  - ➢ Enviserectomy (perforating the foetal abdomen).
  - ➢ Cleidotomy (cutting the clavicles).

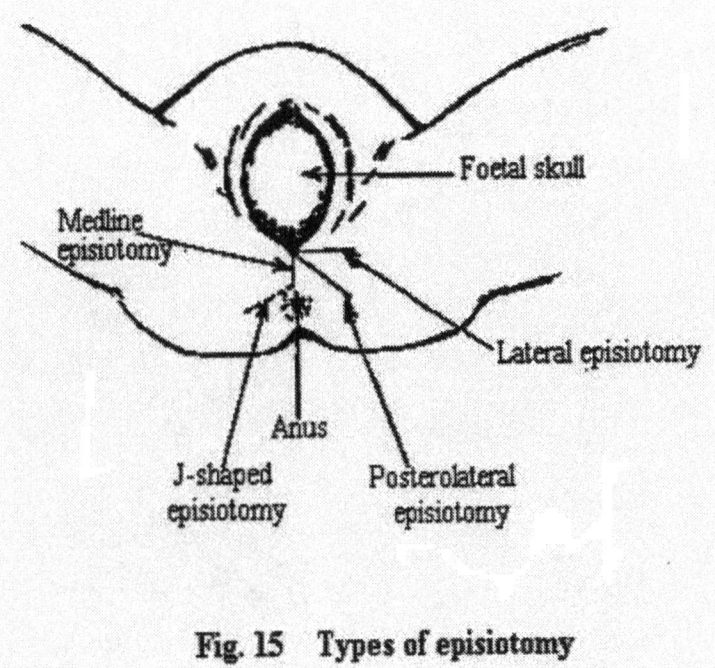

**Fig. 15   Types of episiotomy**

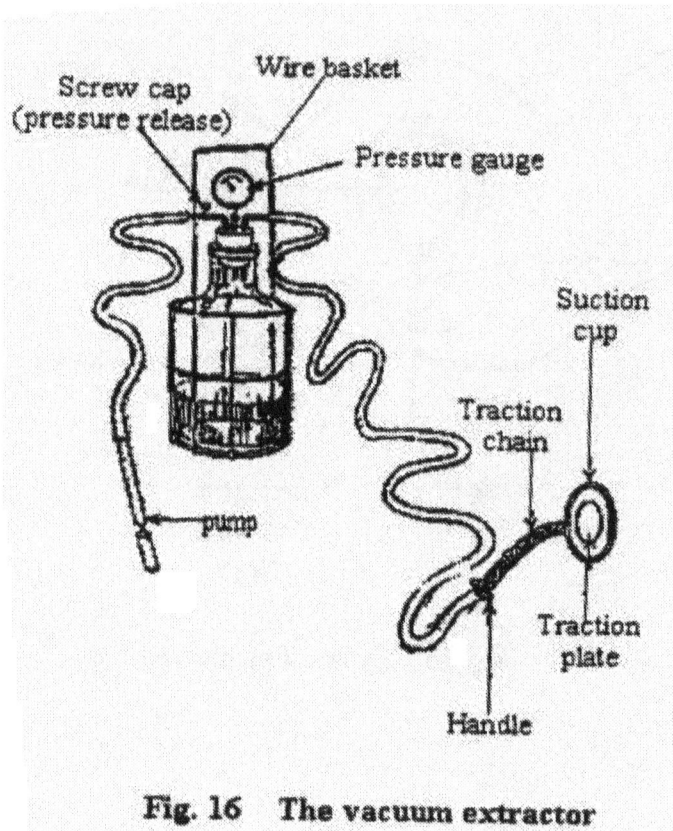

**Fig. 16    The vacuum extractor**

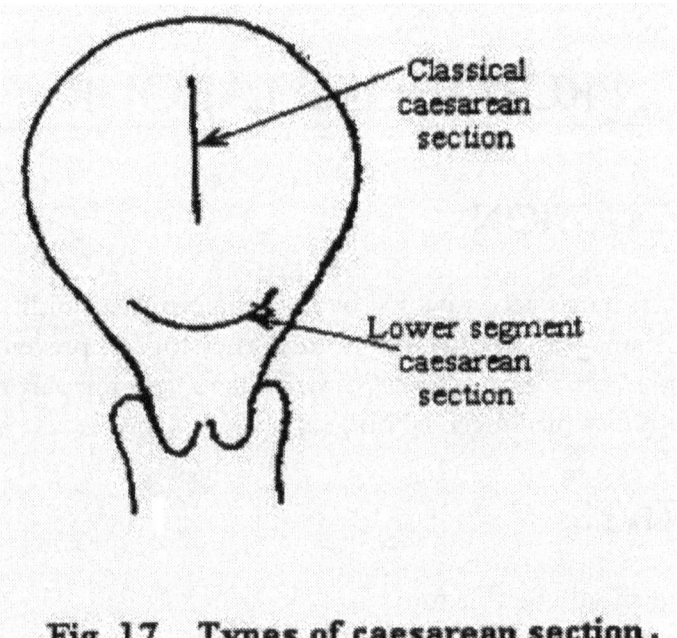

**Fig. 17   Types of caesarean section.**

# CHAPTER 18

# PROLONGED LABOUR

## INTRODUCTION

Prolonged labour is accompanied by high maternal morbidity/mortality. Proper management of labour is the cornerstone of preventing prolonged labour. A Clinical Officer/Midwife has a very big part to play in the prevention of prolonged labour.

## OBJECTIVES

The student should be able to:
- Define prolonged labour.
- List the causes of prolonged labour.
- Predict patients at risk of getting prolonged labour.
- Make a proper observation of a patient in Trial of labour.
- Prevent prolonged labour.
- List the complications of prolonged labour.
- Prevent retention of placenta.

## DEFINITION

Labour is said to be prolonged if it goes beyond 24 hours in both primigravidae and multigravidae. The old saying, "the sun should not set twice on a woman in labour," holds water. In practice, as many women come into the hospital when already in established labour, the principle in our labour ward is that such a woman should be delivered within 12 hours.

> A WOMAN WHO IS IN ESTABLISHED LABOUR SHOULD BE DELIVERED WITHIN 12 HOURS.

# CAUSES OF PROLONGED LABOUR

The causes of prolonged labour may be the same for both the first and the second stages of labour.

The causes of delayed first and second stage labour can be considered under the 3 P's:

- Faults in the passage.
- Faults in the passenger.
- Faults in the powers.

## Faults in the passage

The passage is the maternal pelvis. There are different types of pelvises.

- Gynaecoid pelvis. This is the normal female pelvis. The transverse diameter of the pelvic inlet in a gynaecoid pelvis is longer than the antero-posterior diameter (see chapter on Obstetrical Anatomy). In East African women a small gynaecoid pelvis is a common type of abnormality. The old term for this type of pelvis was "East African pelvis". Such a small pelvis may lead to obstruction of the passage of the baby at the pelvic brim.
- Anthropoid pelvis. In this pelvis the antero-posterior diameter is longer than the transverse diameter. Anthropoid pelvis predisposes to occiput posterior position in vertex presentation. This pelvis may lead to delayed second stage of labour.

- Android pelvis. This is the male type of pelvis. The brim pelvis is roughly triangular. This pelvis may cause obstruction of labour at any level or point of the pelvis.
- Flat pelvis. In this pelvis the transverse diameter is longer than the antero-posterior diameter. Usually obstruction of labour occurs at the inlet.
- Other pelvises include those with flat sacrum, deformed pelvis due to infection (polio and tuberculosis), pelvic bony tumours and fractures of the pelvis.

## Diagnosis of contracted pelvis

- A contracted pelvis is likely in a woman with previous history of abnormal deliveries, prolonged labour, instrumental deliveries or caesarean section.
- Skeletal system deformity especially of the spine and pelvis.
- A woman who is 145 cm or less tall is likely to have contracted pelvis.
- Short pelvic diameters (see chapter on obstetric anatomy).

Management of patient with contracted pelvis will be discussed in the chapter on Trial of Labour.

## Faults in the passenger

The passenger is the foetus. The faults of the passenger can be:
- Malpresentation like face, shoulder, brow or compound presentation.
- Abnormal lie like transverse and oblique.
- Malposition of vertex presentation like deflexed head and occiput posterior.

- Abnormal parts of the foetus like hydrocephalus, swellings of the neck and abdomen (due to ascites or renal tumours, enlarged liver or spleen).

## Faults in the powers

The powers are the uterine contractions. During labour normal uterine contractions begin simultaneously in the region of the insertions of the round ligament, the so called "pace maker". Uterine contractions spread from the pacemaker to the whole uterus. This is called "polarity". The contractions are strongest at the fundus of the uterus and become gradually weaker and of shorter duration the further down they go towards the cervix. During contractions the uterus feels hard and painful while in between contractions the uterus feels soft and not painful. There are about three types of abnormalities of uterine contractions.

- Weak uterine contractions. The uterus may be hypotonic or go into inertia. This type of abnormal uterine contraction occurs especially in primigravidae. The uterine contractions are of normal polarity but they are abnormally weak and infrequent. Prolonged labour usually results. The uterine inertia can either be primary or secondary.
  - ➢ Primary uterine inertia occurs more in primigravidae than in multigravidae. This inertia starts from the beginning of labour and thus the progress of labour is very slow. The abdominal pain is minimal and the contractions are weak thus both the mother and the foetus remain normal with little danger to either unless membranes are ruptured. In such inertia if membranes are intact they should be ruptured and contraction may start to be strong. If membranes are ruptured and inertia still continues augment labour with Syntocinon (see 'Induction of Labour'). If despite augmentation of labour, contractions are

not getting stronger, rule out pelvic disproportion and such patients should be referred to hospital.

➢ Secondary inertia is essentially due to uterine exhaustion or uterine muscle fatigue. Secondary uterine inertia can occur during the first, second or third stages of labour. If this inertia occurs in the first or second stages of labour rule out pelvic disproportion, malpresentation, malposition or ruptured uterus (especially in multigravidae). During secondary inertia the woman develops electrolyte imbalance, dehydration and acidosis. Such patients with secondary uterine inertia should be infused with 5% Dextrose intravenously and referred to hospital with relatives to donate blood if operation is going to be resorted to. Uterine inertia during the third stage labour needs to be managed actively (see chapter on 'Normal Labour'). If the placenta can not be delivered quickly the patient should be referred to hospital with an intravenous drip of Normal saline or dextrose-saline.

• Excessive uterine contractions. Excessive uterine contractions commonly occur in obstructed labour especially in multigravidae, injudicious use of oxytocin during stimulation of labour or some " traditional " medicines used to stimulate labour may have an oxytocic effect. The complications of excessive uterine contraction include foetal death and uterine rupture (especially in multigravidae).

> **THE UTERUS OF A PRIMIGRAVIDA DOES NOT RUPTURE WITH EASE UNLESS TRAUMATIZED.**

Patients with excessive uterine contractions should be referred to hospital for if the contractions do not get reverted, caesarean section may be necessary.

• Abnormal polarity of uterine contractions.

➢ Hypertonicity of the lower segment.

➢ Reversed polarity.

➢ Local or generalized tonic contractions.

Such uterine contractions are painful but not productive. Foetal distress is common in these types of abnormal uterine polarity. Such patients should be sedated and referred to hospital for delivery as caesarean section may be necessary.

- Cervical stenosis due to fibrosis may prevent the cervix from dilating.

# COMPLICATIONS OF PROLONGED LABOUR

The following complications can occur due to prolonged labour.

- Obstructed labour. If prolonged labour due to pelvic disproportion or malpresentation is allowed to go on for too long, it reaches a point of obstruction. In multigravida the uterus continues to contract until it ruptures and then stops contracting where as in primigravidae the uterus goes into secondary uterine inertia. Obstructed labour can lead to vaginal fistula (especially in primigravidae).
- Infection. Before labour the uterine cavity is protected from infection by the closed cervix, cervical mucus plug, and the intact amniotic membranes. In prolonged labour, especially if membranes are ruptured, infection is common within 24 hours. The infection may lead to poor uterine contractions, infect the baby in utero and spread into pelvic organs and lead to puerperal sepsis.
- Maternal and foetal distress (see later).
- Postpartum haemorrhage. Patients with prolonged labour should be referred to the hospital immediately as they can end up with post-partum haemorrhage.

## Prevention of prolonged labour

Prolonged labour can be prevented by:
- Selecting, during antenatal period, the high risk patients for obstructed labour. Such patients to should be referred to hospital early before they go into labour.
- All high risk patients to stay near or in hospital from 37 weeks of gestation until delivery. The suggestion of having maternity villages near a hospital is worth trying in developing countries.
- Anaemia should be corrected in all high risk patients as many might need some operative delivery.
- Labour should be supervised by the use of PARTOGRAM (see chapter on Partogram).
- Patients with 'Poor Progress of Labour' should be referred to hospital as soon as possible.

# PROLONGED THIRD STAGE OF LABOUR

Traditionally the third stage is said to be prolonged, delayed or retained, if the placenta is not delivered within one hour. With active management of the third stage of labour any placenta undelivered within 30 minutes is unlikely to be delivered spontaneously thereafter.

## Causes of retained placenta

There are many causes of retained placenta:
- Mismanagement of the third stage of labour (see under chapter on Normal Labour). This is the commonest cause!
- Morbid adherence of the placenta.
  - ➢ Placenta accreta.
  - ➢ Placenta increta.
  - ➢ Placenta percreta.
- Uterine atony.

## Management of retained placenta

A patient with retained placenta should be referred to hospital immediately whether she is bleeding per vaginum or not.

A PATIENT WITH RETAINED PLACENTA CAN DEVELOP PPH WHETHER SHE IS BLEEDING VAGINALLY OR NOT.

Such a patient should have a drip of normal saline running and should be sent with donors as she might need blood transfusion. In the hospital the placenta should immediately be delivered manually under anaesthesia, by a doctor. The manual removal of the placenta should not be delayed for the excuse that blood for transfusing the patient is not available.

FURTHER DELAY OF DELIVERING THE PLACENTA WILL WORSEN THE PPH.

AN EMPTY.CONTRACED AND UNINJURED UTERUS DOES NOT BLEED.

The patient should be given antibiotics before and after manual removal of the placenta.

## Prevention of retained placenta

Except for the morbid adherent placenta active management of the third stage is the secret for the prevention of retained placenta. Even Traditional birth attendants (TBAs) are afraid of retained placenta.

THE BATTLE IS NOT OVER UNTIL THE PLACENTA IS COMPLETELY DELIVERED.

# POSTPARTUM HAEMORRHAGE (P.P.H)

Postpartum haemorrhage can be either primary or secondary.
- Primary postpartum haemorrhage is defined as bleeding per vaginum in excess of 500 mls of blood occurring within the first 24 hours from delivery. Postpartum haemorrhage is one of the three common causes of maternal mortality in many developing countries. Other common causes of maternal mortality are sepsis and eclampsia. Primary PPH is sometimes divided into two.
  - ➤ Third stage PPH. This is the bleeding occurring before the placenta is delivered.
  - ➤ True PPH. This is the bleeding which occurs after delivery of the placenta.
- Secondary PPH. This is the PPH occurring after 24hours of delivery up to end of puerperium.

## Causes of PPH

- The causes of primary PPH include:
  - ➤ Retained placental tissues (cotyledons or membranes) or blood clot.
  - ➤ Uterine atony.
  - ➤ Laceration of the genital tract as in uterine rupture, cervical tears, perineal tears and episiotomies.
  - ➤ Bleeding disorders.

> AN EMPTY CONTRACTED AND UNINJURED UTERUS DOES NOT BLEED.

- Possible causes of secondary PPH include:
  - ➤ Retained placentae tissues or blood clot. The retained tissues will invite an ascending infection.
  - ➤ Chorionic carcinoma (see chapter on trophoblastic disease).

# Treatment of PPH

All patients who have developed PPH in a health centre should immediately be referred to hospital. Before referring the patients try to get the cause of the PPH and assess the patient's condition. If the condition can be treated at the health centre treatment should be done without delay, unless the patient's condition is too bad. It is imperative to set up an intravenous infusion and let it run fast.

- In the third stage PPH the placenta should be removed. At the health centre the midwife should try to rub up a uterine contraction and apply fundal pressure to deliver the placenta or try controlled cord traction. If the above trials are not fruitful the patient should be referred to hospital where these methods will be tried, failure of which, the placenta could be removed manually under general anaesthesia.
- In true PPH.
  - ➤ The placenta should be inspected to rule out retained cotyledons or membranes.
  - ➤ The genitalia should be inspected to rule out perineal tears. The anterior vaginal wall should be inspected as even small tears in this area can cause heavy vaginal bleeding.
  - ➤ The uterine should be and explored digitally to rule out blood clots and retained placental tissues.
  - ➤ If the uterus is empty but not contracting it should be massaged abdominally.
  - ➤ If bleeding still continues despite the said efforts the following should be done.
    - ✓ Catheterise the urinary bladder and empty any urine.
    - ✓ Bimanual compression of the uterus.
  - ➤ If bleeding persists the patient should immediately be referred to hospital where the said methods will be tried or hysterectomy may be resorted to.

- In secondary PPH. A Syntocinon drip should be set up. Ergometrine 0.5 mg. intravenously is given stat. If bleeding continues the patient should be transferred to hospital where digital examination of the uterine cavity or gentle uterine curettage will be done. In persistent P.P.H. hystorotomy may be resorted to.

## Complications of PPH

More women die due to PPH than during pregnancy, first stage, and second stage of labour and puerperium. The main complications of PPH include:

- Anaemia.
- In severe PPH the woman can go into hypovolaemic shock and even death.

> IN AN ANAEMIC PATIENT EVEN A SMALL BLOOD LOSS MAY LEAD TO PPH.

- Infection. An anaemic woman can succumb to infection with ease due to lack of immunity. The main infections are bacterial and protozoal. The patient can easily become septicaemia.
- Sheehan's syndrome. This is ischaemic necrosis of the anterior pituitary gland. The involvement of the anterior pituitary gland may lead.
  - ➢ Amenorrhoea.
  - ➢ Infertility due to failure to ovulate.
  - ➢ Intolerance to heat.
- Hypofibrinogenaemia. Due to loss of blood the serum fibrinogen level will also be reduced.

## Prevention of PPH

All efforts should be done so as to prevent PPH. The prevention should be done both during the antenatal period and at delivery.

- During antenatal period.
  - ➤ Anaemia should be treated vigorously.
  - ➤ Patient at risk of developing PPH should be identified and manage properly. Patients at risk of developing PPH include those with:
    - ✓ Previous history of PPH.
    - ✓ Previous history of retained placenta.
    - ✓ Bleeding tendencies.
    - ✓ Multiple pregnancy.
    - ✓ A.P.H.
- Managing the third stage of labour actively.

# CHAPTER 19

# TRIAL OF LABOUR

## INTRODUCTION

Trial of labour is a common procedure done in hospitals. The midwife will be expected to conduct such a delivery.

## OBJECTIVES

The student is expected to be able to:
- Define trial of labour.
- List the pre-requisites for trial of labour
- Manage a woman under trial of labour.

## DEFINITION

Trial of labour is one of the methods of managing cephalo-pelvic disproportion (CDP). Other ways of managing CDP are elective caesarean section or induction of premature labour. Trial of labour is the method recommended in all patients suspected to have CDP. It is recommended when there is borderline pelvis. The hope is that with the degree of giving (stretching of the pelvic ligaments), overlapping of the foetal head, strength of uterine contractions and degree of flexion of the foetus, vaginal delivery may be achieved.

# PRE-REQUISITES FOR TRIAL OF LABOUR

- Trial of labour should only be done in a place where caesarean section can be done immediately, if called for.

TRIAL OF LABOUR SHOULD NOT BE DONE IN A HEALTH CENTRE.

- The presentation of the foetus should be vertex; any other presentation is contraindication for trial of labour. Occiput-posterior position is not a contraindication for trial of labour.
- There should be no other obstetric high risk factor like previous caesarean section, diabetes mellitus and heart disease.

# MANAGING A PATIENT UNDER TRIAL OF LABOUR

- The theatre staff should be informed about the procedure so as to get ready in case labour is terminated.
- The patient should take nothing orally as she could go for caesarean section at anytime. A drip of 5% dextrose should be put up and run slowly.
- The progress of labour should be monitored closely by the use of partogram.
- The foetal heart rate should be monitored quarter hourly and maternal blood pressure and pulse be recorded hourly.
- Labour should be terminated (trial of labour is said to have failed) if one of the following conditions develops.
  - ➤ Failure of progress of labour in the presence of good uterine contractions.

> ➤ Failure of the cervix to dilate any more or the cervix becoming oedematous.
> ➤ Failure of the presenting part to descend or considerable caput or moulding of the foetal head.
- Maternal distress.
- Foetal distress.

# CHAPTER 20

# OTHER ABNORMALITIES
# OF LABOUR

## INTRODUCTION

Other abnormalities of labour to be discussed are as important as prolonged labour.
Some of these abnormalities may even occur along with or as a complication of prolonged labour.

## OBJECTIVES

The student should be able to diagnose, manage and prevent the following conditions.
- Foetal distress.
- Premature rupture of membranes.
- Pre-term labour.
- Precipitate labour.

## FOETAL DISTRESS

Foetal distress occurs when placental circulation or exchange of nutrients is sufficiently disturbed so as to produce changes in the foetal heart rate and muscle tone. The major insult in foetal distress is hypoxia (foetal asphyxia) leading to foetal acidosis. Initially hypoxia gives rise to foetal tachycardia but as it gets worse, foetal bradycardia and arrhythmia set in. The accumulation of carbon dioxide ($CO_2$), increased hypoxia, acidosis and hypercarponea (hypercarbia) lead to parasympathetic .stimulation of the gastro-intestinal tract and relaxation of sphincter ani. The relaxation of the sphincter ani results in the passage of meconium by the foetus.

If the asphyxial insult is not removed promptly, foetal death occurs or if the baby is born alive it will suffer brain damage.

## Clinical features of foetal distress

The diagnosis of foetal distress depends on certain clinical signs, bio-physical and biochemical tests:
- Meconium staining of liquor. Expect in breech delivery where meconium staining is common, due to squeezing of the foetus, stained liquor denotes foetal distress, either acute or chronic. The amniotic fluid can be observed after rupture of membranes, amniocentesis (aspirating the amniotic fluid with syringe) or amnioscopy. The amniotic fluid is greenish if meconium stained. The muconium can be graded into:
  - ➤ Grade I. This is light coloured staining of liquor.
  - ➤ Grade II. This is between grade I and III.
  - ➤ Grade III. This is thick, 'Pea soup' like.
- Alteration of foetal heart beat. Normal foetal heart beat is 120–160 beats per minute. The foetal heart can be fast (tachycardia) rate above 160 beats per minute or slows (bradycardia) rate below 120 beats per minute. An irregular foetal heart-beat within the normal range is normal. The rhythm and regularity of the foetal heart can be monitored by a cardiotocogram machine that

can monitor foetal heart rate and rhythm, and uterine contractions continuously. As such a machine is only available in big centres; the midwife may have to depend on the monoaural foetal stethoscope. The foetal heart should be monitored continuously for at least one minute during and after contractions. The possible foetal heart rhythms are:

➤ Deceleration or Type I dip deceleration (early deceleration). The foetal heart decelerates with uterine contraction but regains its normal rate immediately after the contraction. This Type I dip is a normal behaviour of the foetal heart.

➤ Bradycardia (tachycardia) or Type II dip (late deceleration). The foetal heart decelerates with uterine contraction but it takes time to regain its normal rate after contraction has stopped. Type II dip is common in uteroplacental insufficiency.

➤ Variable deceleration is common in cord compression.

• Foetal blood pH can be done in well developed centres with astrup machines that can analyse the foetal blood pH, oxygen and carbon dioxide. The blood is taken from the foetal scalp. Foetal blood pH below 7.2 indicates foetal acidosis.

• Low apgar score. Usually a foetus which is distressed is born with a low apgar score (see under Care of the Newborn).

## Management of foetal distress

Management of foetal distress is largely empirical while waiting for delivery and or transfer of patient to hospital. The midwife in the health centre should resuscitate the foetus by:

• Nursing the patient on her side so as to avoid supine hypotensive syndrome.

• Administer high concentration of glucose intravenously so as to increase glucose supply to the foetus.

- Membranes should be ruptured if still intact. The liquor will be meconium stained. If the liquor is clear most probably the foetus is not in distress.
- Oxytocin, if it is being used, should be stopped.
- Monitoring the foetal heart more frequently, after every five minutes. In centres with cardiotocogram machine, continuous foetal heart monitoring should be done.
- Making preparation to resuscitate the baby after delivery (see Care of New-born).
- Making preparation to deliver the woman. The baby must be delivered by the quickest and fastest method. If the foetal distress is detected during late second stage of labour, vacuum extraction can be applied to deliver the baby, if this is feasible. If the foetal distress is diagnosed during the first stage of labour the patient should be referred to hospital, immediately, for caesarean section. The patient should be escorted by a well equipped trained midwife.

## Causes of foetal distress

Foetal distress is an expression of a decrease in uterine, placental and or cord blood flow, plus nutritional deprivation; especially in placental insufficiency, leading to foetal hypoxia and acidosis. Foetal distress can be acute, chronic or additive.

- Causes of acute foetal distress.
  Acute foetal distress is that distress which arises suddenly, for the first time, during pregnancy, labour or delivery. The major causes of acute foetal distress include:
  ➢ Marked reduction in foetal circulation or placental perfusion. This is so in umbilical cord accidents (cord prolapse, true cord knots), hypertonic uterine contractions naturally occurring or

induced by injudicious use of oxytocin/prostaglandins), maternal hypoxia and abruptio placenta.

➢ Inadequate systemic circulation as in shock, sudden heart failure, placenta praevia, foetal cardiac failure (hydrops foetalis), myocarditis, foetal congenital abnormality of the heart and cord.

➢ Inadequate blood oxygenation due to severe maternal anaemia and haemorrhage, foetal acute haemolytic crisis (Erythroblastosis foetalis), impaired respiratory efforts (as in tetanus and acute poliomyelitis), hypoxia, and or hypercarbia in poorly controlled anaesthesia, eclampsia, status epilepticus, status asthmaticus, cardiac arrest and Mendelson's syndrome.

• Cause of chronic foetal distress.

Chronic foetal distress is the distress which starts to operate in the prenatal period. It is usually a result of utero-placental insufficiency caused by several pathological states.

➢ Marked reduction of placental perfusion or foetal circulation. This can occur in PIH, diabetes mellitus, chronic renal disease, postmaturity (post-date), multiple pregnancy (twin-to-twin transfusion competition for circulation) and intrauterine infection.

➢ Inadequate systemic circulation as in acquired and congenital cardiovascular diseases in the mother, foetal congenital cardiovascular anomalies, maternal-foetal transfusion syndrome and accidental injection of anaesthetics into foetal circulation through the placenta during paracervical or caudal block.

➢ Impaired blood oxygenation in extensive tuberculosis, emphysema, impaired respiratory efforts (as in kyphoscoliosis), low oxygen tension (in high altitudes), difficult labour and prolonged labour.

• Additive or combined causes of foetal distress.

> ➤ Acute foetal distress superimposed on chronic foetal distress as discussed earlier.
> ➤ Drug over-dosage.
> ➤ Prolonged use of narcotics.

# MATERNAL DISTRESS

Maternal distress occurs in prolonged labour. The ketoacidosis and electrolyte imbalance which occur during prolonged labour can affect the metabolism and functions of all the muscles of the mother.

## Clinical features of maternal distress

A woman who has developed maternal distress will be:
- Restless and anxious due to lack of sleep and abdominal pains.
- Dehydrated due to loss of fluid both into the gastrointestinal tract and perspiration. Also she loses water by vomiting and thus cannot take in fluids. Her tongue will be dry and furred due to dehydration.
- The pulse rate will be over 100 beats per minute.
- Body temperature may be raised.
- The guts will be distended by gas due to paralytic ileus caused by the electrolyte imbalance.
- The respiration will be rapid and deep due to acidosis.
- Urine output will be reduced and the urine will be concentrated.

## Management of maternal distress

- 5% Dextrose infusion of about 1,500 mls should be administered intravenously and fast so as to rehydrate the patient. 20 mls of 50% glucose should be added to the above drip so as to increase calories. This will prevent patient from utilizing fat for energy.
- Sedation with morphine 15 mg intramuscularly is important.

Usually the above treatment corrects the maternal distress and labour continues. If the above treatment does not improve labour, then labour should be terminated. If the woman is in late second stage, labour can be terminated at .a health centre by performing vacuum extraction. Sometimes if the presenting part of the foetus is at the perineum, a large episiotomy may be all that is needed.

If the patient is in first stage of labour then she should be referred to hospital for possible caesarean section.

## Prevention of maternal distress

- Prevention of prolonged labour is the major way of preventing maternal distress.
- During labour patients should be encouraged to drink plenty of concentrated glucose fluids. For the women who have been restricted to take nothing per oral (for example. those in trial of labour) a 5% dextrose infusion should be given.

# PRECIPITATE LABOUR

Precipitate labour means that the course of labour has been rapid with intense and frequent contraction and delivery has occurred within one hour. Precipitate labour is not common. Precipitate labour can occur physiologically in grandmulitparous women or may be caused by the administration of oxytocin/prostaglandins.

## Complications of precipitate labour

Precipitate labour is dangerous to both the mother and her foetus.
- In the mother. Laceration of perineum and/or cervix is common.

- The foetus is in great danger as it can get asphyxiated in utero due to the tetanic uterine contractions. Intracranial haemorrhage is common as it passes rapidly through the birth canal. The baby many be injured by being delivered in an unsuitable place and/or falling on the floor.

## Management of precipitate labour

- If the baby is already born injuries in both the mother and the newborn should be ruled out. The newborn should be given Vit. $K_1$ intramuscularly to prevent haemorrhage from either occurring or continuing.
- If the baby is not yet born, the mother can be given pethidine 100 mg intramuscularly immediately and referred to hospital under the escort of an equipped midwife. In hospital tocolytic drugs or general anaesthesia could be given so as to stop the contractions.

# PRETERM LABOUR

Preterm labour is defined as labour which starts before 37 completed weeks of pregnancy but above 20 weeks. The babies born usually weigh less that 2500 mg.

## Causes of preterm labour

There are many causes of preterm labour. They are more or less similar to the causes of abortion.

- Febrile illnesses like malaria, urinary tract infection and pneumonia. The fever is the cause of uterine contractions.
- Trauma to the pregnant abdomen.
- Strenuous exercises like walking/travelling long safaris, not getting enough rest even from usual domestic chores.
- Severe anaemia.

- Congenital abnormalities of the uterus, like bicornuate uterus.
- Premature rupture of membranes (PROM), either spontaneously or iatrogenically.
- Uterine fibroids, especially the submucous and the intramural type.
- Cervical incompetence.
- Congenital malformations of the foetus.
- Other pregnancy states like multiple pregnancy, polyhydramnios, antepartum haemorrhage, RH-incompatibility, severe PIH and eclampsia.
- Miscalculated dates where by the pregnancy is induced for fear of being overdue.

## Management of preterm labour

Management of preterm labour depends on whether the labour is established or not.

- If the labour is established, that is inevitable (whereby the cervix is dilated 4 cm or more, uterine contractions are strong, and/or membranes are ruptured) then labour is going to continue thus the midwife should be ready to resuscitate the preterm baby. The delivery of the baby should not be traumatic. The second stage should be assisted so that the foetal head does not come out fast. An episiotomy makes the delivery of the head smooth. Fast delivery of the foetal head can cause cerebral haemorrhage. The born preterm baby and its mother should be referred to hospital for care.
- If labour is not established, expectant management should be instituted. The mother should be referred to hospital where the cause, if detected, is treated.

The patient could be given tocolytics so as to counteract uterine contractions). If the pregnancy is less than 32 weeks of gestation the patient should be given Dexamethasone 12mg intramuscularly 12 hourly for 24 hours so as to mature the foetus' lungs. Sexual intercourse should be avoided for some time as it can cause or worsen uterine contractions.

## Foetal complications of pre-term labour

Preterm labour, if not stopped, will result in a preterm baby being born. A preterm baby is a baby born before 37 weeks of gestation but above 24 weeks of gestation. The baby born will weigh less than 2500 gm. There are many complications that a preterm baby can get:
- During delivery the baby can get cerebral trauma leading to cerebral haemorrhage.
- After delivery the baby can suffer from Respiratory distress syndrome (RDS) as their respiratory centres are still immature. The babies can get:
  - Hypothermia due to immature temperature regulating centre.
  - Jaundice, due to the immature liver.
  - Bacterial infection due to their reduced body resistance.
  - Bleeding tendency.

  Preterm babies need close management.
  - Oral secretions should be sucked.
  - Should be kept warm.
  - Vit. $K_1$ 1.0 mg should be given intramuscularly.
  - Early feeding with glucose is essential.
  - The babies should be isolated so that they do not get infections from other babies or visitors.

## Prevention of preterm labour

Sometimes the cause of preterm labour is not known.

- Pregnant women should be advised to attend antenatal clinic early in pregnancy and regularly so that such conditions as anaemia, PIH and urinary tract infection can be detected and treated at an early stage.
- Pregnant woman should be advised to abstain from heavy physical work and travelling long distances.
- Pregnant women should be given prophylactic antimalarial and haematinics.
- The women at risk of getting preterm labour like multiple pregnancy and polyhydramnios should be referred to hospital early enough for further management.

# PREMATURE RUPTURE OF MEMBRANES (PROM)

Premature rupture of membranes is defined as rupture of membranes before onset of labour. The causes are mostly unknown. PROM can be brought about iatrogenically either during induction of labour or accidentally during membranes sweeping. It is also suspected that a week point in the amniotic membranes could rupture before labour starts. It is common in multiple pregnancy, polyhydramnios and if the presenting part of foetus is poorly fitted into the pelvis.

After premature rupture of membranes labour may set in within 6 hours or the leaking of liquor many continue for days
or weeks or the rupture many close spontaneously.

## Dangers of premature rupture of membranes

- Dry labour. If most of the liquor drains out the foetus will be in close contact with the uterine walls, thus labour will be dry.

- Ascending infection is common after 24 hours. The ascending infection can cause amnionitis, neonatal pneumonia and even peritonitis if the infection spreads. Signs of infection will include smelly liquor, high temperature and pulse rate of the woman and the foetal heart beat will be raised (tachycardia).
- Cord prolapse.
- Abruptio placenta.

## Management of PROM

All women with PROM should be referred to hospital. Before referring such a patient to hospital ascertain that what is coming out per vaginum is liquor and not urine or pus by:

- History. The patient will complain of sudden watery vaginal discharge.
- Investigations.
  - ➤ Odour of the discharge. Urine has ammonical smell, while liquor smells like seminal fluid.
  - ➤ Alkalinity. Liquor is alkaline so it will change litmus paper blue.
  - ➤ Liquor contains vernox caseosa (fat globules).
  - ➤ Liquor contains lanugo hair from the foetus.
  - ➤ Fern test. In liquor fern test is positive. If the discharge is smeared on a microscope slide and examined under microscope it will form a fern-like structure.
  - ➤ Foetal squames. Liquor will contain foetal squames; so if mixed with 0.1% solution of Nile blue sulphate, the foetal squames will appear orange.

The management of PROM depends on the gestation period.

First and foremost cord prolapse should be ruled out. If the cord is pro-lapsed then pregnancy should be terminated regardless of the gesta-tional age. If there is no cord prolapse then:

- If the gestation period is above 34 weeks or above, the dangers of the foetus staying in utero are more than if delivered. Thus at this gestation period the woman should be delivered and care of the baby is done accordingly.
- If the gestation period is less than 34 weeks then conservative management can be tried.
  - ➤ If gestation period is less than 24 weeks salvaging the preg-nancy is not easy.
  - ➤ If there is a lot of liquor draining out salvaging the pregnancy is not easy.
  - ➤ If there is infection the best management is to terminate the pregnancy.
  - ➤ If there is none of the above, conservative management can be tried.
    - ✓ Bed-rest.
    - ✓ Prophylactic antibiotics.
    - ✓ Corticosteorids can be given to the mother so as to mature the baby's lungs. Dexamethasone 12 mg, intramuscularly, 12 hourly for 24 hours.

While on conservative management the maternal pulse and the temperature and the foetal heart rate should be monitored fre-quently. The draining liquor should be smelled every day to detect infection. In hospitals where cultures can be done, frequent cul-turing of the liquor should be done. During conservative manage-ment avoid unnecessary vaginal examinations.

# SHOULDER DYSTOCIA

## Definition

The anterior shoulder of foetus is stuck behind the maternal pubic symphysis and can not be delivered easily.

## Mechanism

The anterior shoulder of the foetus can get stuck behind the maternal pubic symphysis when the bisacromial diameter (the distance between the two shoulders) occupies the anteroposterior plane instead of a slight oblique position of the maternal pelvis (see mechanism of labour in chapter 15).

## Causes

It is not easy to predict the occurrence of shoulder dystocia. There are risk factors.

- Maternal.
  - ➢ Android or anthropoid pelvises.
  - ➢ Diabetes mellitus.
  - ➢ Excessive weight gain.
  - ➢ Obesity.
  - ➢ Multiparity.
  - ➢ Post date or overdue pregnancy.
  - ➢ Prolonged second stage of labour.
  - ➢ Previous shoulder dystocia or macrosomia.
- Foetal.
  - ➢ Large baby.
  - ➢ Macrosomia.
  - ➢ Advanced gestational age.
  - ➢ Increased chest to head ratio.

# Diagnosis

When a gentle downward traction of foetal head fails to accomplish delivery of the infant's anterior shoulder the midwife should suspect shoulder dystocia.

# Management

Shoulder dystocia is a rare obstetrical emergence. Many times there is no time to refer the patient to an Obstetrician. It is therefore very important to train all attending midwives on what to do in this case. If there is an Obstetrician nearby his/her assistance should be sort immediately. Patients with the high risk factors should not be delivered in a health centre. The Obstetrician should be within reach during the delivery of patients with the high risk factors listed above.

As soon as shoulder dystocia is suspected the patient should stop bearing down as the shoulder impaction could be made worse. Urinary bladder should be drained. One of the following manoeuvres should be performed immediately.
- McRobert's manoeuvre.
  This is the most common manoeuvre. The patient's legs are hyperflexed. This causes cephalad rotation of the pubic symphysis and flattening of the lumbar lordosis. This causes disengagement of the baby's anterior shoulder and delivery of the baby can be done. Many times this is all that is needed. If anterior shoulder does not dislodge then suprapubic pressure can be applied to dislodge the impacted anterior shoulder. The pressure may be exerted in a posterior (Mazzanti manoeuvre) or lateral (Rubin) direction to help the bisacromial diameter of the foetal shoulders into the oblique plane.

- All four position (Gaskin manoeuvre).
  The patient assumes the knee-chest position. The midwife stands behind the patient to assist the delivery of the baby.
- Squatting position.
  This is the common position used during delivery by Traditional birth attendants (TBAs) in Tanzania. The patient sits on a stool and supported from the back by an assistant. The midwife sits in front of the patient to assist the delivery.
- Fracture of the clavicle.
  Pressure is applied anteriorly and posteriorly away from the foetal lungs and the clavicle(s) is/are fractured at the distal portion.
- Other less familiar manoeuvres include: Wood screw, Rubin, and Zavanelli.

## Complications of shoulder dystocia

- Foetal injuries.
  - ➤ Brachial plexus injuries due to excessive lateral traction of the foetal head. This can give rise to palsy.
    - ✓ Erb's palsy, if nerves C5 to C6 are damaged.
    - ✓ Klumpke's palsy, if nerves C7 to T1 are damaged.
  - ➤ Clavicular fracture.
  - ➤ Death if there is much delay in delivering the baby.
- Maternal.
  - ➤ Uterine rupture especially in multigravidae.
  - ➤ Injury to the birth canal.
  - ➤ Infection.
  - ➤ Haemorrhage.

# CHAPTER 21

# THE PARTOGRAM

## INTRODUCTION

In Tanzania the MCH-4 form (appendix–1) for screening high-risk women during pregnancy is common in all antenatal clinics. The detection of poor progress of labour can easily be done by the use of a partogram. The partogram has been found in many developing countries to be a cheap and effective method of detecting poor progress of labour. In delivery units where the Partogram is unpopular many women go into prolonged labour at the expense of their own lives and that of their babies. The Ministry of Health of Tanzania is trying to popularise the use of partogram.

## OBJECTIVES

The student should be able to:
- Define partogram.
- Describe the parts of a partogram.
- Record the progress of labour on a partogram, correctly.
- Refer patients to hospital early before they pass the action line of the partogram.

# DEFINITION

The partogram is also known as labour graph or cervicograph. The partogram can be defined simply as a graphical record of the progress of labour.

# PARTS OF PARTOGRAM

The partogram shows the progress of labour, condition of the mother and her foetus. Since the introduction of partogram by Philpot, R.H. and Castle (1972) there have been a lot of modifications of the partogram. The one recommended by the World Health Organisation (WHO) which includes pre-drawn alert and action lines (appendix–3) is the one dealt with in this chapter.

## Progress of labour

The partogram has a portion for monitoring the progress of labour in terms of cervical dilation, descent of the presenting part and strength of uterine contractions.

- Cervical dilation and descent of the presenting part are combined in one graph.
  - ➢ The Cervico-graph. The x-axis denotes hours. Each space in the x-axis is one hour and spans from 0–24 hours. The y-axis is numbered 0–10 which is equivalent to cervical dilation in centimetres. There is a bold horizontal line from 0–8 hours at 3 cm dilation. The horizontal line forms the latent phase of labour. At the 8th hour of the horizontal line is an oblique line drawn diagonally; this is the "Alert line". The Alert line denotes the active phase of labour. An "Action line" is drawn four hours after the alert line and parallel to it.

- Uterine contractions are also presented graphically in terms of the number of contractions per 10 minutes and the intensity; see under recording on partogram.

## Foetal condition

The foetal condition is presented graphically in terms of foetal heart rate, colour of liquor and degree of moulding of the foetal skull bones.

## Maternal condition

The maternal condition is graphically presented in terms of blood pressure, temperature and urine for proteins, acetone and volume.

# RECORDINGS ON THE PARTOGRAM

Before recording on the partogram a good history and examination of the woman should be done so as to establish that is in labour or not (appendix–7). When the patient is found to be in labour then the partogram can be started.

## Recording cervical dilatation

The cervical dilatation is recorded in centimetres though assessed by finger breadth. At admission if the cervix is still less than 3 cm dilated, the dilation is recorded at time o with an x. The date and time are written underneath (appendix–6). The patient is said to be in the latent phase of labour. If the cervix is 3 cm or more dilated, the dilatation is recorded on the alert line in the active phase (appendix–5) and the date and time should be written underneath. The cervical dilatation is usually assessed four hourly until the time of delivery. The cervical dilatation can be assessed earlier than the said time if:

- The amniotic membrane rupture, so as to rule out cord prolapse.

- The patient wants to bear down so as to ascertain that the cervix is fully dilated. If the patient bears down with a partially dilated cervix, the cervix will be oedematous and/or cervical tear.
- If the cervix was 7 cm or more dilated at the last examination.
- If there signs of foetal distress so as to see if the cervix is fully dilated and vacuum extraction can be performed to expedite delivery of the baby.

If the patient was admitted in the latent phase the next cervical assessment, after four hours, may give rise to two possibilities:

> The cervical dilatation may still be less than 3 cm dilated. The dilatation is then recorded at time 4 hours (appendix–4).

> The cervical dilatation may be 3 or more cm dilated. The dilatation is also recorded at time 4 hours, but then transferred to the alert line (appendix–6).

If the patient was in the active phase of labour and the cervix dilates normally (at the minimum rate of 1 cm per hour) the next assessment the cervical curve will be on or to the left of the alert line. If the curve for cervical dilatation is on the right of the alert line then the active phase is getting prolonged.

## Recording descent of the foetal head

The baby's head is arbitrarily divided into five horizontal equal parts. As labour progresses the number of parts (fifths) of the foetal head remaining above the brim is assessed and recorded on the labour graph with a 'o' (appendix 4–6). The number of fifths above the brim is determined by abdominal palpation, hourly. During cervical assessment bimanual palpation can be done to ascertain the number of fifths of the foetal head which are above and below the brim. Vaginal examination alone can be misleading due to caput formation of the foetal scalp. Due to caput formation the foetal head can be at the pelvic outlet while the largest part of head is still above the brim.

If the membranes rupture during labour this should be noted and recorded at the appropriate time. The following abbreviations are used for the rupture of membranes.

- S.R.M. = spontaneous rupture of membranes.
- A.R.M. = artificial rupture of membranes.

## Recording for moulding of the foetal skull bones

Moulding or over-lapping of the foetal skull bones is graded and recorded on the partogram as follows:

- O = Means the bones are normally separated.
- + (1°) = the bones are touching one another but not overlapping.
- + + (2°) = the bones are overlapped but can be separated with ease.
- + + + (3°) = the bones are overlapped so much that they and cannot be separated.

## Recording maternal condition

The maternal pulse and blood pressure are recorded in their appropriate column. Urine, in particular the acetone and protein, is always recorded (appendix–3)

## Other recordings

In the partogram there is a portion for recording drugs and intravenous fluids given to the patient during labour. There is an area particularly for oxytocic therapy for induction or augmentation of labour.

## Short notes

Short notes can be written on the partogram but long notes can be written on the back of the labour graph or on a separate sheet of paper.

# HOW TO MANAGE LABOUR BY USING A PARTOGRAM

The partogram was originally meant for use in primigravida at peripheral clinics. Now the partogram should be used in all wards and for all patients who have been allowed to go into labour and vaginal delivery anticipated.

- If the patient is admitted in the latent phase she should be examined again after 4 hours. If she is still found to be in the latent phase she could be given Pethidine 100 mg intramuscularly. After the pethidine, the patient who is in true labour will continue to have uterine contractions. The patient who continues to be in labour after the pethidine should have A.R.M. done, if the membranes are intact. If after 8 hours the cervix is still less than 3 cm dilated she should be referred to a hospital as she might need augmentation of labour.

- If the patient is in the active phase of labour, cervical dilation should be along or above the alert line. Any patient who crosses the alert line should be referred to hospital. During labour the patient should empty her bladder frequently. If the membranes are intact the patient could be given an enema and ARM could be done later. A patient who crosses the alert line should be referred to hospital before she reaches the action line unless she is about to deliver.

LABOUR SHOULD BE MANAGED ACTIVELY.

- The foetal head is expected to descend simultaneously with the cervical dilatation. In the African woman, at times, the head delays to descent until late in first stage of labour if her pelvis has a high angle of inclination. When the cervix is fully dilated delivery should be effected within one hour, if not second stage of labour is said to be delayed and the patient be referred to hospital immediately. Note that the patient should not be forced to bear down until crowning of the foetal head has occurred.

In hospital the referred patents are again assessed to see why they have crossed the alert line and treated accordingly before reaching the action line. The action line should not be crossed for more than 4 hours before an action of delivering the patient is taken. After the patient has delivered a summary of the labour should be written under the partogram (appendix–3).

# CHAPTER 22

# THE PUERPERIUM

## INTRODUCTION

Traditionally, the puerperium period is the period of rejoicing for the newborn, the mother is well taken care of nutritionally and she is not supposed to do any strenuous work. If pregnancy and labour were managed properly the puerperium period will be with fewer problems. If the woman is mismanaged during the puerperium period, problems like infection and bleeding can occur.

> DELIVERY OF A DEAD BABY DEPRIVES THE PATIENT THE PRIVILEGES OF THE PUERPERIAL PERIOD.

## OBJECTIVES

The student should be able to:
- Define puerperium.
- Describe the normal physiological changes during the puerperium.
- Describe the establishment of lactation.
- Manage a woman in her puerperal period.

# DEFINITION

The puerperium is the period following childbirth. It starts after delivery of the placenta up to six weeks that is, 42 days. Traditionally it takes only 40 days and in some traditions like the Digos of Tanzania, the fortieth day is marked by a ceremony whereby the baby is taken out of the house for the first time. During the puerperium, traditionally, the woman is not supposed to have sexual intercourse. Sexual intercourse, in some traditions, is performed on the fortieth day.

# PHYSIOLOGICAL CHANGES DURING THE PUERPERIUM

During the puerperium period the mother is physiologically returning more or less to her pre-pregnant state. The greatest anatomical changes can be observed in the uterus and the breasts.

## Lochia

Lochia is the discharge from the genital tract after delivery. The lochia consists mainly of blood and necrotic decidua from the uterine cavity. For the first 3 4 days lochia is red (lochia rubra), then change to reddish-brown (lochia serosa) from the 4$^{th}$ to 7$^{th}$ day and thereafter the lochia is yellowish in colour (lochia alba). By the 10$^{th}$ or 14$^{th}$ day the patient should not have an abnormal vaginal discharge.

## Uterine involution

Involution of the uterus means its return to its pre-pregnant state. The involution of the uterus is due to the dramatic withdrawal of the placental hormones. The hypertrophied uterine cells release their excessive fluid by "autolysis". The blood vessels at the placenta area get thrombosed. The endometrium is well regenerated by the 10$^{th}$ to 14$^{th}$ day, except at the placental area where it takes about six weeks.

At the end of the third stage of labour the contracted uterus is at the level of 20 weeks gestation and weighs about 1.0 kg. The uterus involutes rapidly in the first week of puerperium and thereafter involution is slower until end of the puerperium. On abdominal examination involution is at the rate of one finger breadth per day and by the 12$^{th}$ puerperal day the uterus will have sunk behind the symphysis pubis.

## The cervix during the puerperium

Immediately after delivery, the cervix is patulous, flabby, bruised and purple in colour. The internal Os is 3–4 cm dilated. After 48 hours the size and volume of the cervix is diminished and there are no bruises. The internal os is dilated to 1–2 cm and as days go by the cervix gets closed. The cervix does not return to its nulliparous state and its external os has slit(s).

# ESTABLISHMENT OF LACTATION

The breasts are being prepared for feeding during pregnancy. There is glandular and ductal proliferation, mainly due to oestrogen and progesterone, during pregnancy. After delivery the breasts' glandular tissues become very active and the breasts increase in size.

Prolactin, a hormone from the anterior pituitary gland, causes the breast glands to secrete milk. Oxytocin from the posterior pituitary gland acts on the myo-epithelial cells surrounding the glands of the breast and causes milk to be secreted into the ducts of the breast and hence into the nipple. The oxytocin also stimulates the output of more prolactin

No matter how far the breast is developed during pregnancy, milk is never produced until the placenta is delivered or ceases to function. The placental oestrogen inhibits the release of prolactin from the pituitary gland. Immediately after inhibition is removed, the outflow of prolactin initiates lactation.

Lactation, that is milk production, is maintained by suckling or stimulation of the nipple, which causes secretion of prolactin. The actual delivery of the milk from the nipple is brought about by the action of the oxytocin on myo-epithelium.

The secretion of oxytocin is in response to nipple stimulation causing the "let down reflex". This let down reflex explains why suckling or fondling of breast causes strong contractions of the puerperal uterus which are also known as "after pains". Oxytocin can also be released by psychological stimuli like the cry of a baby or when the mother is getting ready to feed her baby.

Colostrum is the secretion produced by the breast during the first three days of puerperium. The production of colostrum is under the influence of oestrogen. Colostrum is yellowish in colour and contains epithelial cells from the breast's glands. Colostrum has high quantities of antibodies which the baby requires during the first month of life.

> COLOSTRUM IS GOOD FOR THE NEWBORN BABY SO MOTHERS SHOULD BE ENCOURAGED TO BREASTFEED AS SOON AS POSSIBLE AFTER DELIVERY.

# MANAGEMENT OF THE PUERPERIUM

In the past women were observed in the postnatal ward for at least seven days. Nowadays women are sent home within 24–48 hours after a normal delivery. Such discharged women should be seen at the postnatal clinic after six weeks or earlier if there are any problems. Before the end of the puerperal period the care of the woman is still the responsibility of the midwife. Before discharging the mother, she should be educated so that she knows normal and abnormal symptoms of puerperium.

## The abdomen

Within the first 24 hours of delivery after pains are normal .Persistence of abdominal pains should raise the suspicions of infection or retained blood clots or placental tissues; thus the patient should be examined and treated accordingly before discharge.

## The lochia

Passage of blood clots per vaginum indicates that, the site of the placenta is not involuting properly; this might necessitate use of oxytocin or curetting the uterine cavity. Persistence of bright red lochia for more than 10 days may mean poor involution. The lochia should be less in amount and its colour should fade each day. Lochia should not be offensive; such state indicates infection. The woman who notices any abnormality of lochia should report to clinic as soon as possible.

## The breasts

The breasts should be prepared for feeding even during pregnancy. Inverted nipples or infected breasts should be treated quickly. Engorgement of breasts is due to incomplete emptying of the breasts. Engorged breasts are tender and hot and the woman may feel febrile.

- If the baby is dead the breasts should not be expressed. The patient should be given analgesics like aspirin. Milking down the breast will encourage more milk production and further breast engorgement. Stilboestrol should not be used as it can cause thrombin-embolism, which is more dangerous than breast engorgement.
- If the baby is alive express the milk manually and let the milk be fed to the baby until it can suck by itself

# CHAPTER 23

# DAMAGE TO THE GENITAL TRACT

## INTRODUCTION

Damage to the genital tract is very common during delivery. Some of the damages can be dangerous if not diagnosed and treated early.

## OBJECTIVES

The student should be able to:

- List the common parts of the female genitalia which can be damaged during labour.
- Diagnose the different genital parts damaged.
- List the causes of genital tract damage.
- Manage, properly, a patient with damaged genital tract.
- Manage a patient with previous caesarean section.

## COMMON TYPES OF GENITAL TRACT DAMAGE

The perineum, vagina, cervix and the uterus can all be damaged during labour and delivery.

236

# PERINEAL AND VAGINAL TEARS

There are three degrees of perineal tears.
- First degree perineal tear is damage to the skin to the fourchette but not involving the muscles.
- Second degree perineal tear is a stage where the posterior vaginal wall and perineal muscles are torn at varying degrees. In severe form the sphincter of the anal canal is damaged and the patient may be incontinent of flatus and/or faeces.
- Third degree perineal tear is the tear which has extended and opened the anal canal. The tear may extend up to the rectum.

## Causes of perineal and vaginal tear

The possible causes of perineal and vaginal tears include:
- Rapid delivery of the foetal head.
- Delivery of a big baby.
- Extraction of the posterior shoulder.
- Narrow pubic angle of the pelvis. This forces the foetal head to find space posteriorly.
- Delivery of persistent occiput-posterior position (face to pubis) of vertex presentation.
- Breech delivery without performing episiotomy.
- Vacuum or forceps delivery without performing episiotomy.

## Repair of perineal and vaginal tears

The first degree perineal and vaginal tears do not need repair unless there is a bleeding vessel. Tears of the upper vaginal wall bleeding profusely should be repaired. The repairing of the second degree tear is like repairing an episiotomy (see chapter on operative delivery).

> **REPAIRING AN EPISIOTOMY IS EASIER THAN REPAIRING A TEAR.**

Third degree tears and severe second degree tears should be repaired under general anaesthesia.

The repairs should be done as soon as possible. A tear not repaired after 24 hours is definitely infected. Repair of an infected tear will not be successful. An infected tear should not be repaired until infection has subsided and the tear edges well healed.

## Prevention of perineal and vaginal tears

- The foetal head should be delivered slowly.
- Care should be taken during delivery of the posterior shoulder.
- A generous episiotomy should be performed in high risk patients and those with signs of impending perineal tear.

The junction between the upper and lower segment forms an oblique line running just below the umbilicus. The sulcus so formed is called the pathological ring or Bandl's ring. When the bandl's ring is formed, rupture of uterus is imminent. In primigravida the uterus goes into inertia during obstructed labour thus it is essentially immune to spontaneous rupture.

- Operative delivery.
    - ➢ Destructive operation.
    - ➢ Forceps delivery.
- Old caesarean section scar.
- Internal podalic version.
- Use of oxytocin/prostaglandins, particularly in grand multiparous.

## Diagnosis of uterine rupture

- Women at High risk of uterine rupture include:
  - ➤ Multigravidae.
  - ➤ Previously scarred uterus for example caesarean section, cornual pregnancy, hystorotomy and myomectomy especially if the uterine cavity had been entered.
- Symptoms.
  - ➤ Sudden pain in the suprapubic area.
  - ➤ Restlessness.
- Signs.
  - ➤ Bandl's ring.
  - ➤ Cessation of labour pains, as the uterus stops to contract.
  - ➤ Vaginal bleeding.
  - ➤ The foetal parts may be easily palpable as the foetus is usually extruded out of the uterus into the peritoneal cavity.
  - ➤ The foetal heart stops as the foetus usually dies.
  - ➤ Pulse rate increases due to reduced blood volume.
  - ➤ Blood pressure is usually low due to blood loss.
  - ➤ Patient becomes pale due to loss of blood.
  - ➤ Abdomen distends.
  - ➤ Tender abdomen with rebound tenderness.
  - ➤ Cold sweat due to hypovolaemic shock.

## Management of ruptured uterus

If the patient delivers quickly at the health centre, explore the uterine cavity manually immediately after delivery of the placenta, to rule out uterine rupture. If no rupture is detected the patient should be observed in the postnatal ward for at least 48 hours before discharging her. The observation at the postnatal ward should include monitoring the blood pressure and pulse hourly, looking for any increased vaginal bleeding and tenderness of the abdomen. If any of the aforesaid parameters is getting worse, refer the patient to hospital since there might be an undetected rupture.

If the patient is not yet delivered, refer her quickly to hospital, even if the uterus is impending to rupture. If the patient is shocked, counteract the shock with intravenous fluids available e.g. normal saline. Sedate the patient with Pethidine or Morphed before transfer. The patient should be escorted by a trained nurse and blood donors for the treatment of such a patient will be surgical, either repair of the uterus or hysterectomy, depending on which will be faster. If the uterus is going to be repaired, bilateral tubal ligation is done at the same sitting.

> A PATIENT WHOSE UTERUS IS RUPTURED SHOULD NOT BE LEFT FERTILE.

## Prevention of rupture of uterus

The Clinical Officer/Midwife should be in the fore front to prevent uterine rupture as this condition is associated with high maternal mortality and/or morbidity and 100% perinatal death. Some preventive measures that a Clinical Officer could take at his/her health centre include:

- Early referral of woman at high risk of uterine rupture to hospital for delivery.

- Preventing prolonged/obstructed labour by use of partogram.
- Looking for early signs and symptoms of impending uterine rupture and referring the patients quickly to hospital.
- Use oxytocic/prostaglandins for induction/augmentation of labour, cautiously.
- Proper use of operative delivery instruments.

# CHAPTER 24

# CARE OF THE NEWBORN BABY

## INTRODUCTION

Care of the newborn baby is a team work which involves both parents and the midwife. In the past, the first week of the puerperal period was spent in the hospital, but nowadays women are discharged from hospital within 24 hours after a normal delivery. Therefore, the care of the baby is in the hands of the midwife in the first 24 hours after delivery thereafter the responsibility is put to the mother at home. The mother should therefore be taught how to take care of her baby at home during these 24 hours!

## OBJECTIVES

The student is expected to be able to:
- Take care of the newborn at birth.
- Resuscitate a newborn baby.
- Take care of the neonate.
- Advise mother on the importance of breast feeding.
- Manage abnormal lactation.

# CARE OF THE NEWBORN AT BIRTH

The first fifteen minutes are very crucial. If the baby is asphyxiated in the whole of this period, brain damage is possible. The delivery room should be warm. As soon as the foetal head is delivered excessive mucus should be removed form the baby's mouth.

The baby's oropharynx should immediately be sucked with mucus extractor to remove any secretions. As soon as the baby is born the degree of asphyxia assessed by using the APGAR SCORE" (see table below) within the first minute then after 5 minutes.

# APGARSCORE

| SIGN | 0 | 1 | 2 |
|------|---|---|---|
| Skin colour. | Blue or pale. | Body pink extremities blue. | Whole body pink. |
| Respiratory efforts. | Absent. | Weak or sluggish. | Good strong cry. |
| Muscle tone. | Limp. | Some flexion. | Active motion. |
| Reflex, irritability | None. | Grimace response. | Cry. |
| Heart rate. | Absent. | Slow $< 100$ | Fast $= 100$ |

Score:
- 7–10..............no or slight asphyxia.
- 4–6...............moderate asphyxia.
- 0–3...............severe asphyxia.

Immediately after delivery of the baby it should be held head down so as to encourage drainage of the amniotic fluid from the lungs. After the pulsations of the cord have stopped the cord is clamped with two artery forceps 6 cm from the umbilicus and cut between the artery forceps with sterile scissors. Two tight ligatures then applied on the remaining piece of cord, about 3 cm from the umbilicus of the foetus and the redundant piece of cord cut off. If the baby is asphyxiated the shortening of the cord should be left until after resuscitation of the baby.

## Resuscitation of an asphyxiated newborn

The ABCs of resuscitation should be aimed at. These are A = establish clear airway, B = initiate breathing and C = maintain circulation.

The baby should be put on a warm Resuscitare If there is no such a facility the baby is put head down on a flat board inclined at 30°. The board should be above the attendant's chest height. A light bulb (100 watts) should be over the board to provide heat to the baby. The baby should be dried thoroughly. Mucus should be sucked out, first from the mouth then the nose and trachea.

- If the baby breathes out spontaneously check for the heart rate.
  - If the baby's heart rate is above 100 beats per minute then evaluate the skin colour.
    - ✓ If the skin is pink or there is only peripheral cyanosis the baby should just be observed and monitored.
    - ✓ If the skin is blue the baby should be given oxygen by positive pressure ventilation (PPV) using an ambu bag.
  - If the baby's heart rate is below 100 beats per minute the baby should be treated as stated below.
- If the baby does not breathe spontaneously or is gasping the baby should be intubated and given 100% oxygen using an ambu or

intermittent positive pressure ventilation (IPPV). The heart rate should be checked.

➢ If the heart rate is below 60 beats per minute then cardiac massage should be done.

➢ If the heart rate is between 60–100 beats per minute.
   ✓ If the heart rate is not increasing cardiac massage should be performed.
   ✓ If the heart rate is increasing then ventilation should be continued.
   ✓ If the heart rate is above 100 beats per minute spontaneous respiration should be watched and if it occurs the ventilation can be discontinued.

➢ If the heart rate is below 80 beats per minute after 30 seconds of IPPV the baby should be medicated.
   ✓ Naloxone 0.1 mg/Kg body weight intravenously, through the umbilical cord, to counteract the effect of morphia or pethidine if any of these drugs had been given to the mother within four hours before delivery.
   ✓ 20 mls of 10% Dextrose intravenously so as to counteract hypoglycaemia.
   ✓ 4 mls of 8.4% sodium bicarbonate to counteract acidosis.
   ✓ 1.0 mg of Vit. $K_1$ intramuscularly to prevent bleeding.

Note that resuscitation should not be done for more than 15 minutes. Continuing to resuscitate a severely asphyxiated baby for more than 15 minutes is just going to increase the number of babies with cerebral damage.

---

CARE OF A CHILD WITH CEREBRAL DAMAGE IS VERY EXPENSIVE AND FRUSTRATING.

# Examining the baby

After resuscitating the baby should be examined thoroughly from head to toe.

- General examination.
  - ➢ The head.
    - ✓ Caput succedaneum that is oedema under the scalp.
    - ✓ Cephalohaematoma that is collection of blood under the scalp.
    - ✓ Anterior fontanelle. Bulging anterior fontanelle indicates increased intracranial pressure. The increased pressure may be caused by cerebral haemorrhage.
    - ✓ Ears for any abnormalities.
    - ✓ Head circumference. The average head circumference of a normal newborn is about 34 cm.
  - ➢ Face.
    - ✓ Eyes. Puffiness of the eyes which is common after birth and can stay for one or two days. Sub-conjunctival haemorrhage may be present usually disappears spontaneously without treatment.
    - ✓ The mouth and lips to rule out cleft palate or cleft lip.
  - ➢ Neck. Rule out any abnormalities like swellings and webbed neck.
- Systemic examination.
  - ➢ Respiratory system.
    - ✓ Breathing pattern.
    - ✓ Grunting.
    - ✓ Air entry to the lungs.
  - ➢ Cardiovascular.
    - ✓ Position of the heart.
    - ✓ Heart rate
    - ✓ Heart murmurs.

  ✓ Peripheral blood vessels.
➢ The abdomen.
  ✓ Rule out any abnormal masses or enlarged spleen, liver and kidneys.
  ✓ Rule out exomphalous.
  ✓ The umbilical cord especially the number of its blood vessels.
➢ Musculo-skeletal system.
  ✓ The skin. Looking for paleness haemangomas, petechial haemorrhage and rashes.
  ✓ Movements of limbs.
  ✓ Deformities of the feet and hip dislocation.
  ✓ Extra digits.
  ✓ The Spine-to rule out spine-bifida.
  ✓ Rule out imperforated anus.
➢ Genitalia.Rule out ambiguous sex. If the baby is a male check the urethral opening and the scrotum for testes.
➢ Central nervous system.
  ✓ Moro reflex.
  ✓ Rooting.
  ✓ Stepping.
• Weigh the baby. The average weight of a Tanzanian/Guyanese baby is 3.4 kg. All babies, born alive or dead, should be weighed.

---

**A NEWBORN BABY SHOULD BE EXAMINED THOROUGHLY AND ANY PATHOLOGY EXCLUDED BEFORE HANDING THE BABY TO THE MOTHER.**

# CARE OF THE NEONATE

The neonatal period is that period within the first 28 days from birth. Early neonatal period is the first one week from birth. As stated above, most normal women and babies are sent home within the first 24–48 hours after delivery; therefore, the midwife should take advantage of the 24 hours to teach the mother how to take care of her baby.

## Care of the baby at birth

After resuscitating and examining the newborn baby as described earlier, keep the baby warm. The baby should be wrapped with a baby blanket to keep warm. If the mother is not exhausted and the baby is normal, keep the baby with the mother.

THE MOTHER IS A SAFER INCUBATOR.

If the mother is exhausted keep the baby in a baby cot. If the baby is preterm, transfer both the baby and the mother to a hospital. The pre-term baby may need to be kept in an incubator.

## Care of the cord

The baby's cord should not be dressed. The cord should be cleaned daily with spirit until it drops off. The cord usually dries and drops off between the fifth and tenth days after delivery. The cord can be painted with gentian violet or iodine daily.

POWDERING OR DRESSING THE CORD SHOULD BE DISCOURAGED.

## Discharging eyes

Pus discharge from the eyes of the newborn is always abnormal. The commonest cause of the discharge is infection with gonococci giving rise to "Gonococcal Ophthalmia Neonatorum". The baby usually catches the infection from an infected mother as it passes through the vagina. Pus swab from the eyes should be taken for gram's stain or be sent to hospital for culture and sensitivity. The treatment of gonococcal ophthalmia neonatorum is either application of silver nitrate drops or tetracycline eye drops daily until the infection clears.

## Bathing of newborns

After birth wipe clean the baby. Bathing babies immediately after birth may make them get cold. The vernox caseosa helps to keep the baby warm and it usually disappears on its own.

VERNOX CASEOSA IS NOT A DIRTY MATERIAL.

Later on the baby can be wiped with a hand towel soaked in 1:200 savlon or hibitane. Antiseptics used to clean the baby should not get into the baby's eyes. Later on the baby can be bathed using warm water and wiped dry.

## Feeding the baby

The baby should be put on to the breast to start sucking right after delivery if the mother feels strong and the baby is normal. Breast feeding enhances involution of the uterus by stimulating it to contract through the release of oxytocin. The baby should be put to breast after every 2–3 hours. Note that newborn babies sleep most of the time (20 hours) so the mother baby should wake up the baby to feed.

## A HUNGRY BABY CRIES MORE OFTEN.

If the mother is not feeling well the baby should be given supplement feeds in the first 24 hours. The baby should be given 5% Dextrose; thereafter the baby is given expressed breast milk (E.B.M). The amount of feeds given should be small but frequent (20–30 mls after every three hours). The average feeds should be 160–180 mls/kg body weight per 24 hours. The feeds should be given by spoon or through a naso-gastric tube if the baby is very sick. Bottle feeding should be discouraged.

## TO ENHANCE BREASTFEEDING THE BABY SHOULD ROOM IN WITH THE MOTHER.

## HOSPITALS SHOULD BE BABY FRIENDLY.

To the mother, breast feeding provides psychological satisfaction, prophylaxis against developing cancer of the breast and contraceptive effect.

## BOTTLE FEEDING SHOULD BE DISCOURAGED.

To the baby, breast milk is good nutrition containing all nutrients needed and in the right amount. Milk is clean and sterile. The colostrum contains antibodies to bacterial and viral infections: thus, it protects the baby.

## BREASTFEEDING BABIES DO NOT GET DIARRHOEAL ATTACKS WITH EASE AS THOSE USING BOTTLE FEEDING.

Breast milk is better and safer than milk supplements. Breastfeeding is contraindicated in the following situations.

- Infected nipples. If the infection is on one nipple the baby can be allowed to suckle the normal breast.
- Mastitis. If the infection is on one breast the baby can be allowed to suckle the normal breast.
- Drugs. Drugs like coumarine, antineoplastics, tetracycline, amphetamines, chloramphenical and cimetidine if taken by the mother are secreted in the milk and have a negative effects on the baby. These drugs should not be used by a breastfeeding mother. If the mother has to use these drugs then she should not breast-feed her baby.

# PROBLEMS OF LACTATION

Problems of lactation could be due to the mother or baby. Problems of lactation due to the mother could be due to:
- Flat or inverted nipples. If the mother has flat or inverted nipples the baby cannot suck the breast properly. During pregnancy invert or flat nipples should be pulled out. The patient should be taught how to pullout the nipples by using fingers or a nipple sucker. After delivery if the nipples are still flat or inverted the mother should express the milk by hand and give the baby the expressed milk.
- Sore nipples. Sore nipples during lactation are caused by the baby biting the nipple with the gums due to bad breast feeding techniques. The nipples get cracked and breast feeding becomes painful. During this painful period the mother should take the baby off the breast and feed her with EBM. Usually the nipples heal spontaneously. When the nipples have healed the mother should be taught how to put the baby on the breast correctly. The baby's gums should bite behind the nipples on the areola of the breast during breast feeding.

- Infected breasts. Mastitis and breast abscess may follow a sore nipple. The mother should be given antibiotics, and if there is an abscess, incision and drainage of the abscess should be done. The baby should continue to suck from the normal breast. The milk from the infected breast should be expressed and thrown away.
- Breasts not producing enough milk (milk insufficiency). The cause of milk insufficiency is mainly due to inadequate breast emptying, psychological or chronic disease like tuberculosis. The mother should be encouraged to take plenty of fluids and eat balanced diet. Worried mothers should get psychotherapy and encouragement.

## Problems of lactation due to the baby

Problems of lactation due to the baby could be due to:
- Preterm.
- Blocked nose.

The baby cannot empty the breasts completely. The breasts will be engorged and milk production reduced. Treatment depends on whether the baby is alive or dead. If the baby is alive encourage the mother to express the breast manually and give the baby E.B.M. Encourage the other to breast-feed frequently. If the baby dead, inhibit lactation as follows.

> The mother should not express the breast as breast engorgement stops milk production.
> Give the mother analgesics, for engorged breasts are painful. Note that the use of stilboestrol should not be practised as it may cause thrombo-embolism and/or withdrawal bleeding. If drugs have to be used bromocryptine or clomiphene can be used but the patient should be told about the chances of ovulating while using these drugs. The traditional empirical measures of inhibiting or suppressing lactation by binding the

breast, giving the mother laxatives, fluid restriction or flooding the cardio-vascular system with fluids are useless.

## Re-establishment of lactation

Lactation can be re-established or improved by:
- Sucking the breast. If a non-lactating woman puts a baby to her breast, frequently, she will eventually start to lactate.
- Good nutrition and fluids to the mother improves lactation.
- There are drugs like prolactin, oxytocin, reserpine, contraceptive pills and phenothiazines such as chlorpromazine which can make a woman lactate.

# CHAPTER 25

# ABORTIONS

## INTRODUCTION

Abortions account for 55% of causes of bleeding in early pregnancy; other causes being ectopic pregnancy and trophoblastic diseases. Abortions account for over 60% of gynaecological admissions in Tanzania and Guyana. Abortion is an important condition not only because of the loss of a baby, if wanted, but because of high chances of maternal death due to haemorrhage and sepsis.

## OBJECTIVES

The students should be able to:
- Define abortion.
- Discuss induced abortion.
- Prevent criminal abortion.
- List the causes of spontaneous abortion.
- Discuss and manage the stages of abortion.
- Diagnose and manage abortion due to cervical incompetence.
- List complications of abortion.

# DEFINITION

Abortion is defined as expulsion of pregnancy before 24 weeks (20 weeks in developed countries) weeks of gestation. Abortion is sometimes known as miscarriage. The abortion can either be induced or spontaneous.

# INDUCED ABORTION

Induced abortion is that abortion in which pregnancy was terminated intentionally. There are two types of induced abortion; criminal abortion and therapeutic abortion.

## Criminal abortion

Criminal abortion is abortion that was induced without any medical indication. In Tanzania, induced abortion is prohibited and considered criminal by law, except on very limited medical conditions. Both the abortionist and the one to whom the abortion is done are considered criminal by law. It is estimated that about 20% of all abortions admitted in Tanzania consultant hospitals are criminally induced. The number of criminal abortions is higher in cities, big towns and urban areas than rural areas (author's observation). The types of women who resort to criminal abortion are:

- Schoolgirls, who are the majority. The schoolgirls resort to criminal abortion because they fear being expelled from school and scolded by their parents, relatives and peer groups.
- Single women for fear of not getting support or being scolded by friends. The women also fear the possibility of not getting married in future.

- Illegitimate pregnancy. Extramarital/out of wedlock pregnancies are not uncommon; but when such misfortune happen over 90% of the women resort to criminal abortion.
- Failure of contraception. Rarely such women resort to abortion as many tend to accept the pregnancy.

> SUSPECT CRIMINAL ABORTION IN A YOUNG UMARRIED WOMAN WITH AN ABNORMAL VAGINAL BLEEDING AND FEVER.

In Guyana termination of pregnancy is legal.

## Complication of Criminal abortions

Criminal abortions are accompanied by many complications including:
- Severe vaginal bleeding which is many times incomplete evacuation of the foetus or injury to the genital organs.
- Injury to the genital organs including perforation of the fornices and/or uterus and tearing the cervix. Genital injuries are common as many of the abortionists are ill-trained on gynaecological procedures.
- Infections. Bacterial infections are very common as, frequently, the instruments used and the places where the abortions are carried out are not sterile.

> IN A PATIENT WITH INCOMPLETE ABORTION WHO IS FEBRILE AND/OR HAS AN OFFENSIVE VAGINAL DISCHARGE CRIMINAL ABORTION SHOULD BE SUSPECTED.

- Menstrual disturbances due to pelvic infections.
- Infertility either due to pelvic infections giving rise to tubal blockage or damage to the uterus and cervix.
- Chronic abdominal pains due to adhesions.

## Management of patient with criminal abortion

Refer all criminal abortions to hospitals. The patient should be resuscitated according to her general state.

- Heavy doses of broad spectrum antibiotics like ampicillin, flagyl and gentamycin, parentrally. The antibiotics are given whether there are signs of infection or not.
- In hospital the patient is examined under general anaesthesia to rule out perforation or injuries to genital organs. The pregnancy should be terminated after 24 hours of the antibiotics whether there are signs of infection or not. Before terminating the pregnancy the cardio-vascular system is loaded with high doses of antibiotics so as to prevent spread of bacteria.

## Prevention of criminal abortion

The case fatality rate and morbidity due to criminal abortion is very high. Prevention is most important. Some of the preventive measures include:

- Family life education to all school girls and boys.
- Emphasize good moral behaviour to adolescents.
- Discourage adolescents from watching pornographic films and videos.
- Allowing adolescents to go to discos should be discouraged.
- Discourage boys and girls from involving themselves in sexual relationships before marriage.
- Educate the public on the dangers of criminal abortion.
- Provide contraceptives to sexually active unmarried girls.
- The girls who fall victim to unwanted pregnancies should not be punished by the state or community. Means should be devised so that such girls after delivery could continue with whatever acceptable activities they were engaged in before.

# THERAPEUTIC ABORTION

Therapeutic abortion is an induced abortion done on medical grounds. There are both maternal and/or foetal indications:

- Foetal indications are all those conditions which make the foetus not survive in utero. Examples include hydrops foetalis, anencephaly or rubella infection. In Tanzania due to lack of diagnostic equipment the foetal conditions warranting therapeutic abortion are not easily detected.
- In assisted fertility 'selective abortion' can be done when there are too many embryos.
- Maternal indications are those that jeopardize the mother's health. Examples include severe hyperemesis gravidarum, cardiac diseases, severe PIH and eclampsia.

Therapeutic abortion should be done by gynaecologists as this procedure is not 100% safe.

## Methods of termination of pregnancy (TOP) include

- Dilatation of cervix and curetting of the uterine cavity (D&C). The D&C can be done for pregnancies which are below 12 weeks of gestation.
- Suction, by use of suction syringe, can be done in pregnancies which are below 12 weeks. This method is safer than D&C.
- Medical induction with either syntocinon or prostaglandins can be done at any gestation.
- Hystorotomy. This is a minor caesarean section. It can be performed for pregnancies which are above 12 weeks in which medical induction has failed.

# SPONTANEOUS ABORTION

Spontaneous abortion is that abortion which occurs without being induced.

## Maternal causes of spontaneous abortions include

- Febrile illnesses. The high temperature induces uterine contractions. Any febrile condition can cause abortion for example malarial infection (commonest), urinary tract infection and pneumonia.
- Trauma either directly onto the abdomen like falling down, kicks; or indirectly like strenuous exercise like walking long distances and travelling.
- Stressful states either psychological (like death of a relative) or physical (like strenuous exercise).
- Chronic diseases like diabetes mellitus and tuberculosis.
- Other infections bacterial, viral, protozoal or treponemal.
- Congenital malformations of the uterus (like bicornuate or septate uterus) or cervix (like cervical incompetence).

## Foetal causes include

- Chromosomal abnormalities. This is the commonest cause of abortion before 12 weeks of gestation.
- Congenital foetal abnormalities like anencephaly and central nervous system like meningocele major.
- Multiple pregnancy.
- Dead foetus.

# STAGES AND TREATMENT OF ABORTION

- Threatened abortion. In this stage the patient complains of mild lower abdominal pains and/or slight vaginal bleeding. The cervix is closed and the products of conception are intact. The patient should be advised to have bed rest either in hospital or at home. The patient can be given sedatives like phenobarbitone or pethidine daily so as to keep her resting. The patient should abstain from strenuous exercises including sexual intercourse, for awhile. If uterine contractions do not cease despite the above treatment then tocolytic drug such as salbutamol can be prescribed. If the cause of threatened abortion is discovered than specific therapy should be given.
- Inevitable abortion. In this stage the patient is going to abort what so ever. The patient usually complains of severe abdominal pains and vaginal bleeding. The cervix is dilated but the products of conception are not expelled. The recommended treatment is to enhance the process of abortion with syntocinon or prostaglandins. Due to severe pains the patient should be sedated.
- Incomplete abortion. In this stage the products of conception are partially expelled. The vaginal bleeding and abdominal pains are usually severe. The cervix is open. The bleeding and abdominal pains may be minimal if only very small pieces of products of conception are remaining in utero. The treatment of incomplete abortion is evacuation of the uterus; therefore, refer the patient to hospital as soon as possible. Before referring the patient, it is important to resuscitate her with intravenous fluids and/or blood, depending on the degree of shock.
- Complete abortion is diagnosed when all products of conception have been expelled. In such an abortion there are no abdominal pains or vaginal bleeding and the cervix is closed. Such a diagnosis before the gestation period of 12 weeks is often incorrect as

frequently small parts of products of conception are left in utero; such patients will continue to bleed, though in small amounts.

> AN EMPTY CONTRACTED AND UNINJURED UTERUS DOES NOT BLEED.

# SPECIAL TYPES OF ABORTIONS

## Missed abortion

See under intra-uterine foetal death.

## Habitual/recurrent abortion

A woman is said to be a habitual aborter if she aborts three or more times, consecutively. In such a woman the cause of abortion is mostly recurrent too. Such a patient should be referred to hospital during or even before the next pregnancy for thorough examination and investigation. Routine investigations for such patients include:

- White blood cell count and differential to rule out infections like tuberculosis.
- Haemoglobin.
- Renal function tests mainly blood urea, creatinine and urine specific gravity to rule out renal diseases.
- Urinalysis to rule out urinary tract infection.
- Fasting blood sugar to rule out diabetes mellitus.
- Blood grouping and Rhesus factor to rule out RH-incompatibility.
- Syphilis tests to rule out syphilis.

Patients with habitual abortion should be treated for the cause if discovered. If the cause is not detected, the patient should be advised bed rest until past the danger period.

## Recurrent late abortions

Recurrent late abortion is a type of habitual abortion occurring from 12 or more weeks of gestation. There are three possible causes:
- Cervical incompetence is the commonest cause (see later).
- Congenital malformation of the uterus for example septate uterus.
- Syphilis. If a pregnant woman is syphilitic her foetus usually dies at 20 weeks of gestation and the baby is expelled later.

## Abortion due to cervical incompetence

Cervical incompetence is the most common cause of recurrent late abortion. An incompetent cervix has a weak sphincter mechanism of its internal os. The possible causes of cervical incompetence are:
- Congenital malformation of the cervix. Such a cervix has few connective tissues thus it cannot hold up a pregnancy. Other causes include a short cervix (less than 2 cm) and if the mother had been using DES (Diethyl stilboestrol) during pregnancy.
- Acquired abnormality of the cervix due to:
  - ➢ Injudicious dilatation of the cervix during D&C.
  - ➢ Cervical cone biopsy after Manchester repair.
  - ➢ Annular detachment of the cervix during obstructed labour.
  - ➢ Old cervical tears.

Clinically patients with cervical incompetence present with the following conditions:
- History of recurrent late abortions.

- The abortion is usually painless. The abortion could be preceded by premature rupture of membranes.
- The abortus could be expelled en bloc.
- The cervix can allow Hegar number 7 when not pregnant. When a Foley's catheter is inserted into the uterus through the cervix and ballooned, if the catheter is pulled it will come out with ease.
- A hystero-gram will be funnel shaped.

A patient with recurrent late abortions should be referred to hospital during or before the next pregnancy for investigation and treatment. The treatment for cervical incompetence is cervical cerclage during pregnancy. The cervical cerclage could be that of Shirodkar or MacDonald types. The cerclage should be applied before 24 weeks of gestation and the earlier it is applied the better. The author applies the cervical suture as soon as he diagnoses the condition, even before 12 weeks of gestation.

PICK THE MANGO BEFORE IT DROPS.

Patients with cervical suture should have strict bed until the pregnancy is 34 weeks.

Cervical cerclage is not without complications; some of the complications include:
- Vaginal discharge due to the foreign suture in the vagina. No antibiotic will dry this discharge thus the patient should be reassured.
- Cervical and/or uterine tear if the patient goes into labour with the suture in-situ. The suture should be removed if patient get uterine contractions which do not respond to tocolytics therapy. The sutures should be removed, routinely, when the pregnancy reaches 37 weeks.

Cervical incompetence, especially the acquired type, can be prevented by:
- Good assistance during delivery so as to prevent cervical tears.
- Prevention of obstructed labour.
- Avoid application of vacuum extractor or forceps when the cervix is not fully dilated.
- Cervical tear should be repaired immediately.
- Proper D&C technique.
- Cervical cone biopsy should only be done in patients who have attained their preferred family size otherwise such patients should be advised to undergo tubal ligation at the same sitting.

# COMPLICATION OF ABORTION

Abortion, whether spontaneous or induced, could have the following complications:
- Vaginal bleeding. If the bleeding is severe it may lead to anaemia, hypovolaemic shock and even death. It is therefore important not to delay treatment of inevitable or incomplete abortion.
- Sepsis is common in criminal abortion and delayed evacuation for incomplete abortion. Clinical features of sepsis include:
  - ➤ Pyrexia.
  - ➤ Increased pulse rate.
  - ➤ Purulent and offensive vaginal discharge.
  - ➤ Tender abdomen.
  - ➤ Tender pelvic organs.
  - ➤ Intestinal ileus.
  - ➤ Leucocytosis.

When sepsis has set in antibiotics in large doses should be prescribed before and after evacuation. The process of evacuation is not without complications.

- ✓ Cervix tear.
- ✓ Perforation of the uterus.
- ✓ Haemorrhage.
- ✓ Sheehan's syndrome.

# CHAPTER 26

# ECTOPIC PREGNANCY

## INTRODUCTION

Ectopic pregnancy is a common gynaecological emergency. Many times patients have ruptured tubal pregnancies. The condition can be fatal if it is misdiagnosed and/or treatment is delayed. Ectopic pregnancy can be tubal, abdominal, ovarian and rarely cervical. Tubal pregnancy will be discussed in this chapter as it is the commonest type of ectopic pregnancies.

## OBJECTIVES

The student should be able to:
- Define ectopic pregnancy.
- List the possible sites for ectopic pregnancy.
- List the causes of tubal pregnancy.
- Refer a patient with tubal pregnancy safely.

## DEFINITION

Ectopic pregnancy is a pregnancy which is implanted outside the uterine cavity.

# SITES OF ECTOPIC PREGNANCIES

The possible sites for ectopic pregnancies include:

- Fallopian tubes. More than 95% of ectopic pregnancies occur in fallopian tubes. Also known as tubal pregnancy. The most common site in tubal pregnancy is the ampulla portion of the tube. Other sites are the isthmus and the interstitial. Tubal pregnancy implanted in the interstitial portion of the tube is also known as cornual pregnancy.
- Abdominal cavity. Also known as abdominal pregnancy.
- Ovary.
- Cervix. Very rare.
- Lesser horn of bicornuate uterus.

# TUBAL PREGNANCY

## Causes of tubal pregnancy

The possible causes of tubal pregnancy include:
- PID. This is the most common cause of tubal pregnancies in Tanzania and many developing countries. The PID causes destruction of the tube.
  - ➤ Tubal blockage.
  - ➤ Destruction of the peristaltic function of the tube. The cilia of the tube, which also helps propel the fertilized ovum, could be destroyed too. Thus a patent tube does not necessarily mean a health tube.
- Infections of the neighbouring organs like appendix (Appendicitis) can lead to pelvic adhesions and thus distortion of the tubes. This is

why tubal pregnancy is more common in the right tube than the left.

- Tumours of the pelvis like uterine fibroids can lead to distortion of the tube.

- Congenital malformations of the tube like small tubular pits or crypts.

## Clinical features of tubal pregnancy

- Symptoms.
  Before rupture of the pregnancy, the symptoms of tubal pregnancy may not be easy to discern. Acute rupture of the tube gives an easy diagnosis, while a slow-leaking ectopic gives rise to a more difficult diagnosis. The symptoms of ectopic pregnancy include:
  - ➢ Amenorrhoea. Usually there is a history of amenorrhoea of 6 8 weeks. In about 5% of the patients there is no history of amenorrhoea.
  - ➢ Abdominal pain. Lower abdominal pain is usual. The pain sometimes radiates to the shoulders due to irritation of the diaphragm by blood.
  - ➢ Vaginal bleeding. The bleeding is usually not heavy. The blood is dark in colour.
  - ➢ The patient may complain of having passed a blood clot but this may be a decidual cast.
  - ➢ Dizziness and fainting episodes due to blood loss.
  - ➢ Retention of urine may develop if a pelvic haematoma develops.
- Signs.
  The signs when the tube has ruptured include:
  - ➢ The patient looks to be in pain.
  - ➢ Tender lower abdomen and/or shocked.

> She looks pale. The paleness is more than the amount of vaginal blood loss.
- The blood pressure may be low and the pulse high and feeble if much peritoneal haemorrhage has taken place.
- On abdominal examination, the abdomen looks distended. The abdomen is tender on palpation with rebound tenderness. Fluid thrill and shifting dullness may be positive.
- On vaginal examination one could find dark blood which is non-clotting. The cervix is closed and excitation sign is positive on the side with the ectopic. One could palpate a cystic tender mass on the involved adnexa. The posterior fornix may be bulging and cystic.

SUSPECT ECTOPIC PREGNANCY IN A WOMAN DURING HER REPRODUCTIVE AGE WHO HAS AN ACUTE ABDOMEN AND IS PALE.

## Aids to the diagnosis of ectopic pregnancy

There are very few aids to the diagnosis of ectopic pregnancy. The aforesaid clinical features should make one suspect ectopic pregnancy. Some aids that can be useful at a health centre include:
- Culdocentesis that is puncturing the pouch of Douglas through the posterior fornix with wide bored needle. The aspiration of dark non-clotting blood indicates haemoperitoneum.
- Abdominal paracentesis through the right or left iliac fossae. The aspiration of non-clotting blood indicates haemoperitoneum. This procedure is not recommended.
- Urine pregnancy test is not very useful.
- Falling haemoglobin. If daily haemoglobin is noted, falling of it indicates continuous blood loss.

- Raised white blood cells count may indicate chronic haemorrhage.
- In a centre with ultrasound, sonography of the abdomen should be performed.
- If the above investigations are inconclusive and the gynaecologist still suspects an ectopic pregnancy a diagnostic laparotomy can be performed or if a laparoscope is available laparoscopy of the abdominal cavity should be done.

## Differential diagnosis

- PID.
- Abortion, in particular the threatened or septic type.
- Any other cause of acute abdomen due to gynaecological or non-gynaecological condition.
- Intra peritoneal haemorrhage due to any other cause like ruptured spleen.

## Management of a patient with ectopic pregnancy

Ruptured ectopic is an emergency condition which need an emergency laparotomy; thus such patients should be referred to hospital without much delay. Before referring the patient quickly resuscitate her with fluids, such as normal saline intravenously, so as to raise the blood pressure. Do not sedate her as doing so may make it impossible for the receiving doctor to elicit some of the important signs like abdominal tenderness. Quickly look for donors to go with the patient. The patient should be escorted by a trained nurse in a comfortable ambulance.

---

UNAVAILABITLITY OF BLOOD SHOULD NOT BE A REASON TO DELAY PERFORMING LAPAROTOMY IN ECTOPIC PREGNANCY.

---

Auto-transfusion during laparotomy can be done and is life saving if the peritoneal blood has not stayed over 12 hours. Infected or haemolysed peritoneal blood should not be auto-transfused.

# CHAPTER 27

# GESTATIONAL TROPHOBLASTIC DISEASE

## INTRODUCTION

Gestational trophoblastic disease is not uncommon in Tanzania or Guyana. The disease is interesting as it raises anxiety in the patient due to its appearance. In some tribes like the Digos in Tanga region, it is believed to be as a result of witchcraft, as the products look like clusters of frog's eggs.

## OBJECTIVES

The students should be able to:
- Define gestational trophoblastic disease.
- List the possible causes of gestational trophoblastic disease.
- Diagnose molar pregnancy.
- Diagnose chorio-carcinoma.
- Reasonable follow up of patients treated for gestational tro-phobastic diseases.

## DEFINITION

Gestational trophoblastic diseases are tumors arising from the trophoblastic layers of chorionic villi.

## CAUSES OF GTD

The causes of GTD are multiple.

- Breakdown to host invader balance. In this state the mother reacts to the genetic elements of her husband during conception. It is for this reason that such diseases are common in first pregnancy.
- Blood group relationship to the couple. If the couple are both blood group "A" then the risk is low. If the female is blood group is "A" and the male is "0" then the risk is high. If the woman's blood group is "AB" she has a high risk of developing the disease with a man of any other group.
- It is common in rice eaters.
- It is common in malnourished and debilitated women.
- It has a geographical distribution. The disease is common in the Far East like Singapore, Malaysia, Hong-Kong and Philippines. The disease is also common in the Middle East. The disease is relatively high in Central Africa and rare in Europe and North America.

## TYPES OF GESTATIONAL TROPHOBLASTIC DISEASE

There are two main types of trophoblastic diseases:

- Hydatidform Mole
- Chorio-carcinoma.

# HYDATIDFORM MOLE

Hydatidform mole is divided into:
- Benign mole which is the typical mole. The mole has all its tissues within the uterus. The mole can change into chorio-carcinoma in 3–7% of the patients. The chances of the mole changing into chorio-carcinoma is greater (10%) in those women aged 40 years or more and those who had three or more deliveries.
- Malignant mole or invasive mole or chorio-carcinoma destruens. This is a locally malignant growth invading the uterine muscles. It can perforate the uterus and be deposited into adjacent organs.
- Metastasising mole. This gives rise to blood deposits commonly to the lungs, vagina, liver and brain. The clinical picture is like that of chorio-carcinoma but histologically they have recognised villous.

## Clinical features of molar pregnancy

- Suggestive symptoms for molar pregnancy include:
  - ➢ Exaggerated symptoms of pregnancy. Hyperemesis gravidarum can be due to molar pregnancy.
  - ➢ Amenorrhoea.
  - ➢ Recurrent brownish or prune like discharge. The patient tends to be admitted in hospital on and off with a diagnosis of threatened abortion.
- Suggestive signs for molar pregnancy.
  The disease becomes clinically apparent or suspected after 12 weeks of gestation. The signs include:
  - ➢ Hyperemesis gravidarum appears in about 12% of patients.
  - ➢ Signs of PIH appear before 20 weeks of gestation.
  - ➢ The uterus is doughy and does not contract.
  - ➢ Foetal parts are not palpated unless there is a co-existing foetus.

> ➤ Foetal heart is not heard as there is no foetus.
- There are signs of thyrotoxicosis due to increased production of thyroxin stimulating hormone (T.S.H.).
- Passage of vesicles is conclusive evidence. The vesicles look like those of hydatids of echnoccocus granulosus. The naked eye appearance of the tumor resembles large branches of grapes or cluster of frog's eggs.

## Investigations for molar pregnancy

The clinical features are important so as to suspect molar pregnancy. Investigations which can be done in a health centre include:
- Pregnancy test. The urine is usually positive for pregnancy test which is due to high production of human chorionic gonadotrophin (H.C.G.) by the tumor. If the urine is positive after being diluted 100–300 times, then highly suspect hydatid-form mole.
- If there are radiological facilities in the health centre an abdominal X-ray can be taken. The X-ray will not show foetal skeleton.
- In a centre with an ultrasound machine sonogram should be done instead of x-ray.

Patients suspected to have molar pregnancy should be referred to hospital where further investigation could be done for example:
- Quantative estimation of H.C.G.
- Angiography.

## Complications of molar pregnancy

The main complications of molar pregnancy include:
- Severe haemorrhage especially during abortion or treatment of the disease.

- Infection especially after abortion; thus the need of prophylactic antibiotics after treating the disease.
- Perforation of the uterus due to the disease itself or iatrogenically during evacuation.
- Change to chorio-carcinoma.

## Treatment of molar pregnancy

The Clinical Officer can do very little in his/her health centre.
- If the mole is expelled spontaneously at the health centre and the patient is bleeding excessively, inject ergometrine 0.5 mg intravenously and perform a digital curettage. This procedure can stop or reduce vaginal bleeding.
- Resuscitate the patient before referring her to hospital.

For the patients referred to hospital:
- If the mole has been expelled spontaneously then a digital curettage is done by the doctor immediately and prophylactic antibiotics given. After three or four days the uterine cavity is curettage with a curette, whether there is vaginal bleeding or not.
- If the mole is not expelled then medical induction with either syntocinon or prostaglandins is done.
- In some centres suction curettage is done under doses of syntocinon or prostaglandins. The traditional dilatation and curettage of the uterus and hystorotomy are outdated.
- In patients at high risk of developing chorio-carcinoma, cytotoxic drugs like methotrexate can be given.

## Follow up

Patients treated for GTD need to be followed up for at least two years. They should be advised not to be pregnant for this whole period.
- HCG monitoring.

➤ Monthly for the first 6months. Pregnancy test should be negative within 8 weeks. If it is ?-HCG it should fall to normal levels within the 8 weeks.

➤ Then every after one month for the next 6 months.

If the HCG continues to be positive or increases in quantity this could be due to:

    ✓ Invasive mole.

    ✓ Metastatic mole.

    ✓ Chorio-carcinoma.

• Chest X-ray. To rule out metastases to the lungs.

➤ Monthly for the first six months.

➤ Then three monthly for the next six months.

When positive this may mean development of metastatic mole or chorio-carcinoma. Skull X-ray should be done when ever the patient complains of headaches and/or develops fits so as to rule out metastases to the brain.

• Liver function test. This should be repeated if it was initially raised.

• Clinical follow up.

➤ Amenorrhoea. When HCG is negative the patient should be expected to get back her menstruation cycles. If the period of amenorrhoea prolongs for more than 6–8 weeks possibilities are:

    ✓ Invasive mole, metastatic mole or chorio-carcinoma.

    ✓ Pregnancy.

    ✓ Hormonal amenorrhoea if she is using hormonal contraceptives.

It is due to above problem that is why the patients should not be allowed to get pregnant for at least two years. She should not use hormonal contraceptives.

➤ Vaginal bleeding. If vaginal bleeding continues after the initial curettage it might mean:
  ✓ Retained products so curettage should be repeated.
  ✓ Invasive mole, metastatic mole or chorio-carcinoma.
➤ Uterine size. Uterine involution should be complete within 6 8 weeks. If the uterus remains bulky this could be due to:
  ✓ Other uterine masses like fibroids.
  ✓ Retained products so curettage should be repeated.
  ✓ Invasive mole, metastatic mole or chorio-carcinoma.
➤ Ovarian cysts. The ovaries might be polycystic due to high levels of HCG.
  When the HCG falls the ovarian cysts usually shrink spontaneously.

# APPENDIX 1

# MINISTRY OF HEALTH
# ANTENATAL CLINIC CARD

| CLINIC: | REG. No. |
|---|---|
| ........................................ | ............................ |
| Name: | Age: .............Height (cm).............. |
| ................................................. | |
| Spouse's name: | Client's Occupation: |
| ............................... | ................................... |
| Ten Cell Leader: | Address: |
| ................................... | |

**PAST DELIVERY**
Gravidity...........                     Parity...............
Abortions..........                      Live babies.........

Date of Last menstrual period (LMP).          Expected date of delivery.
................................................          ..................................

**HIGH RISK FACTORS**
Look for them at first visit.

**A Put (v) where indicated. Refer client to Hospital immediately.**
Age below 16 years..............Delivery of dead baby or Neonatal death.............
Last pregnancy > 10 years.......Three or more consecutive abortions.................
History of previous C/S......... History of Heart disease/Diabetes or TB.............

**B Put (v) where indicated. Refer client to Hospital immediately.**
Eight or more pregnancies..........Age above = 35 years........
Height below 150cm for First pregnancy...............Forceps/Vacuum delivery............
History of PPH..........History of retained placenta.............

Blood group........Rh.............. VDRL.............. Elisa...............
Others...............................

# APPENDIX 1 (CONTINUED)
# NOTE: WRITE CLEARLY

| | | | | | | | | | | | | |
|---|---|---|---|---|---|---|---|---|---|---|---|---|
| Date | | | | | | | | | | | | |
| Weight (Kg) | | | | | | | | | | | | |
| Blood Pressure (mm. Hg) | | | | | | | | | | | | |
| Haemoglobin (gm/dl) | | | | | | | | | | | | |
| Protein in urine | | | | | | | | | | | | |
| Maturity of pregnancy | | | | | | | | | | | | |
| Height/Size of Uterus | | | | | | | | | | | | |
| Presentation | | | | | | | | | | | | |
| Foetal heart beat | | | | | | | | | | | | |
| Antimalarial prophylaxis | | | | | | | | | | | | |
| Ferrous sulphate tabs Folic Acid tabs. | | | | | | | | | | | | |
| Tetanus toxoid | | | | | | | | | | | | |
| **Signature of examiner** | | | | | | | | | | | | |
| Date of next visit | | | | | | | | | | | | |
| Advise on Family planning................. Date..................... She wants BTL after delivery................. Sign of client............ Sign of witness.......... Date..................... | | | | | | | | | | | | |

| Look for these factors always. Put (v) where indicated . Refer to Hospital | | Date and reason for transfer to Hospital |
|---|---|---|
| BP  =140/90 ............ Hb. < 9.0 gm/dl......... Protein in urine......... Pitting oedema.......... Bleeding P.V............ | Pregnancy of > 40 weeks........ Dead baby in utero................ Abnormal lie or presentation of the baby................... Pregnancy or size of the uterus too big/small.................... | Date and reason of Hospital referral.<br><br>Date                    Reason<br>1                          1<br>2                          2................<br>3                          3 |
| Where client to deliver..................... | | Doctors advise later pregnancy ........................................ |

# APPENDIX 2

# WHO IMMUNIZATION SCHEDULE

TT 1: At first contact or as early as possible during pregnancy.

TT 2: At least 4 weeks after TT 1.

TT 3: At least 6 months after TT 2.

TT 4: At least 1 year after TT 3.TT 5: At least 1 year after TT 4 or during the next pregnancy.

TT = Tetanus toxoid.

The WHO is aiming at a Universal coverage (90%) of all pregnant women with at least TT.

(Source: WHO/FHE/MSM/94.11).

# APPENDIX 3

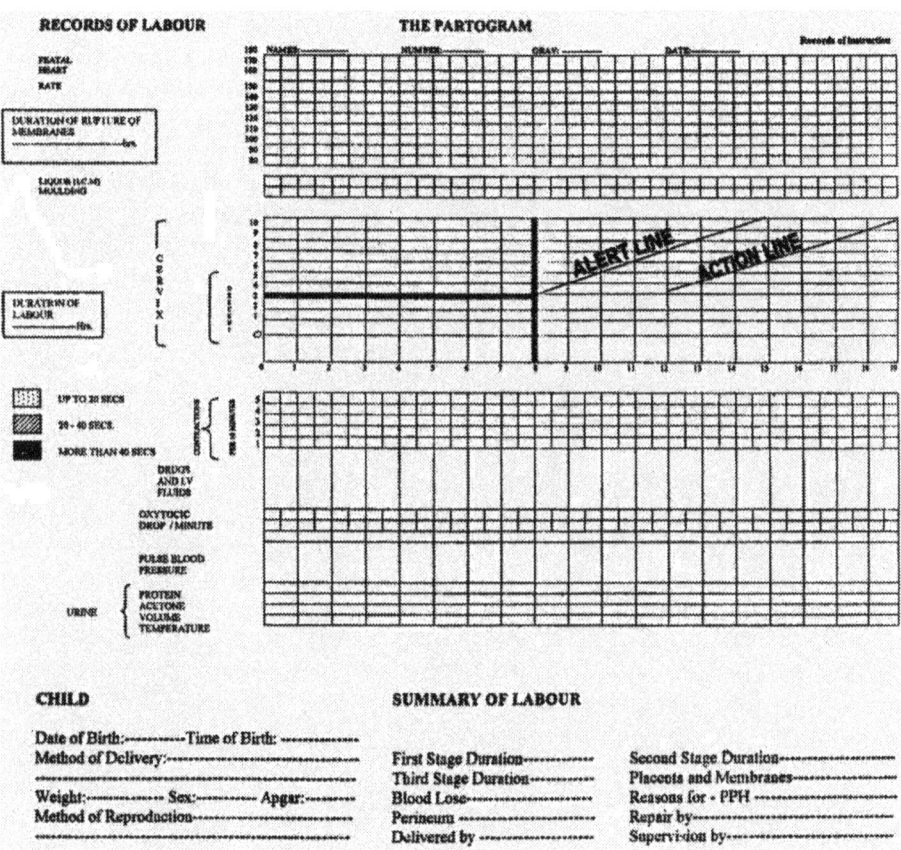

**RECORDS OF LABOUR**

FEATAL
HEART
RATE

DURATION OF RUPTURE OF
MEMBRANES
————————hrs.

LIQUOR (t.C.M)
MOULDING

DURATION OF
LABOUR
————————Hrs.

▦ UP TO 20 SECS

▨ 20 - 40 SECS.

■ MORE THAN 40 SECS

C E R V I X

**THE PARTOGRAM**

NAME: _____ NUMBER: _____ GRAVI: _____ DATE: _____ Records of Instruction

ALERT LINE

ACTION LINE

DRUGS
AND I.V
FLUIDS

OXYTOCIC
DROP / MINUTE

PULSE BLOOD
PRESSURE

URINE { PROTEIN
ACETONE
VOLUME
TEMPERATURE

**CHILD**

Date of Birth:——————Time of Birth: ——————
Method of Delivery:——————————————————
——————————————————————————————————
Weight:—————— Sex:—————— Apgar:——————
Method of Reproduction——————————————————
——————————————————————————————————

**SUMMARY OF LABOUR**

First Stage Duration——————
Third Stage Duration——————
Blood Lose——————————
Perineum ——————————
Delivered by ——————————

Second Stage Duration——————————
Placenta and Membranes——————————
Reasons for - PPH ——————————
Repair by——————————————————
Supervision by——————————————————

283

# APPENDIX 4

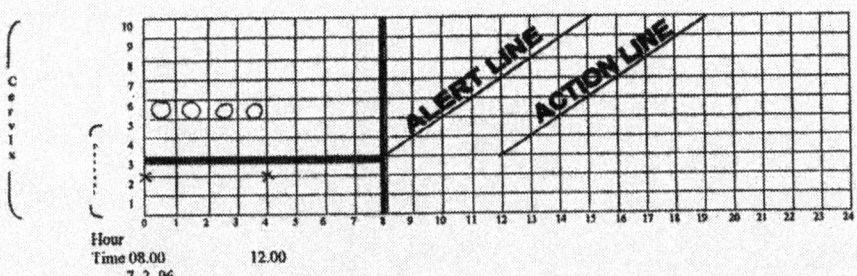

Partogram of a patient admitted in the latent phase at 08.00 am on 7th February, 1996 with cervical dilation of 2cm.
Four hours later she was still in the latent phase with cerival dilation of 2cm. The foetal head was all the time 5/5.

# APPENDIX 5

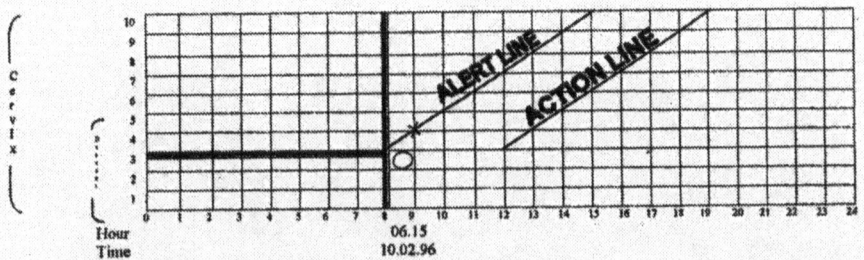

Partogram of a patient admitted in the active phase at 06.15 am on 10th February, 1996 with cervical dilation of 4cm and three parts of the foetal head are below the pelvic brim(2/5).

# APPENDIX 6

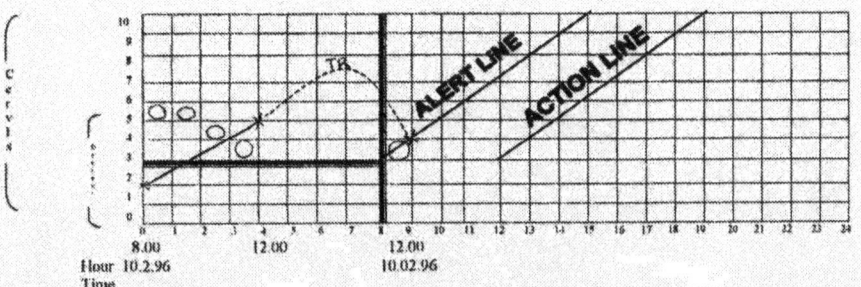

Partogram of a patient admitted in the latent phase at 08.00 am on 10th February, 1996 with cervical dilatation of 2cm and the foetal head at the brim. Four hours later the cervix was 4cm dilated and two parts of the foetal head are below the pelvic brim.

# APPENDIX 7

## RECORD OF LABOUR

Surname.....................
              Other names.................
              Address.....................
              ..............................
              Date of birth
              day......month......year...
              Race.........................
              Tribe...................

Admission date.......................Time...................By whom.......................
Admission (reason of admission etc)..................................................................
From................Home/Hospital transfer/antenatal ward/clinic etc...............................
Summary of Antenatal ...............................................................................
Abnormalities.........................................................................................
      LMP.....................       EDD.....................

Obstetrical history: Gravida...Para..........Living children............

| Year | Maturity | Method | Wt. | Sex | Alive/dead | Complication | |
|------|----------|--------|-----|-----|------------|--------------|--|
|      |          |        |     |     |            |              |  |
|      |          |        |     |     |            |              |  |
|      |          |        |     |     |            |              |  |
|      |          |        |     |     |            |              |  |
|      |          |        |     |     |            |              |  |
|      |          |        |     |     |            |              |  |

Examination:
General condition...................................Fundal Height.....................
Temperature.........................................Size of foetus....................
Blood pressure.....................................Lie..................................
Oedema.............................................Presentation.......................
Urine: Protein..........Acetone....................Foetal heart.......................
Height..............................................Liquor: Membranes intact......
Hb estimation at present...........................Clear.....................
      Last recorded at ANC.......................Meconium stained.......
Blood group.......... Rh............................If membranes ruptured:
                              Date....................
                              Time....................

## INITIAL VAGINAL EXAMINATION AND PELVIC ASSESMENT

Date....................Time........................Examiner...........................

Cervix: State.......... Dilatation...................Bony pelvis (cross which does not apply)

Presenting part.......................................Sacral promontory: Not/ Just/ Easily reached

Level................................................Sacral curve: Normal/Flat

Position..............................................Ischial spines: Normal/ Prominent

Moulding.............................................Sub pubic angle: Normal/ Narrow

Caput................................................Sacral tuberosities: No. of knuckles.

Membranes/Liquor...............................Summary........................................................

Consultant/ Registrar's opinion..............

## BIBLIOGRAPHY

# RECOMMENDED TEXTBOOKS FOR FURTHER READING

A Comprehensive Maternity Nursing: Nursing Process and the Childbearing Family.
>    By: Nelson, Jean D and May, Katharyn.
>    Publisher: J. B. Lippincott Co.

Clinic Gynaecologic Endocrinology and Infertility
>    By: Sheroff, Leon et al.
>    Publisher: Williams and Wilkins Publishers.

Dewhurst's Textbook of Obstetrics and Gynaecology for Postgraduates
>    By: John Dewhurst and D. Keith Edmond.
>    Publisher: Blackwell Scientific Publications.

Fundamentals of Obstetrics and Gynaecology
>    By: Jones Llowylenes.
>    Publisher: Churchill Livingstone Publishers.

Gynaecology Illustrated.
>    By: Govan, Hart and Callender.
>    Publisher: Churchill Livingstone Publishers.

Maternal infant, Nursing care.
    By: Dickson Elizabeth, et al.
    Publisher: C.V Mosby Co.

Medical Disorders in Obstetric Practice
    By: De Swift, Micheal.
    Publisher: Blackwell Scientific Publications.

Myles Textbook of Midwives 2nd Edition
    By: Bennett, Ruth and Brown, Linda.
    Publisher: Church Livingstone Publishers.

Obstetrics Illustrated.
    By: Millers, A and Ballander, A.
    Publisher: Churchill Livingstone Publishers.

Principles of Gynaecology
    By: Jeffcoate, Norman.
    Publisher: Butterworth Publishing Co. Ltd.

# ABOUT THE AUTHOR

Dr. John Naeman Kibiriti Mbilu was born in Tanzania on the 23$^{rd}$ March 1946.

He started his Primary education in 1954. He obtained his degrees of Doctor of Medicine (MD) in 1975 and Master of Medicine (MMed) in Obstetrics and Gynaecology in 1981 from the University of Dar-es-Salaam, Tanzania

He has worked in Tanzanian hospitals from 1975 until 1994. He also worked as a United Nations Volunteer as a Consultant Obstetrician and Gynaecologist, in Guyana and Turks and Caicos Islands from 1994 to 2001 He is now working in St. Lucia as a consultant Obstetrician and Gynaecologist.

Dr. Mbilu has taught Obstetrics and gynaecology to Medical students, Medical Officers students and Midwifery students in Tanzania and Guyana. He was also a Senior Lecturer in the University of Guyana. He has accumulated worldwide knowledge and practical skills in Obstetrics and Gynaecology.

Dr. Mbilu is as a member of the Association of Gynaecologists and Obstetricians of Tanzania (AGOTA), Medical Association of Tanzania (MAT) and Guyana Medical Association (GMA).

0-595-25646-5